The Control of Fertility

THE CONTROL OF FERTILITY

Gregory Pincus

THE WORCESTER FOUNDATION FOR EXPERIMENTAL BIOLOGY
SHREWSBURY, MASSACHUSETTS

1965

ACADEMIC PRESS   New York and London

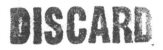

ACADEMIC PRESS INC.
111 Fifth Avenue, New York, New York 10003

United Kingdom Edition published by
ACADEMIC PRESS INC. (LONDON) LTD.
Berkeley Square House, London W.1

LIBRARY OF CONGRESS CATALOG CARD NUMBER: 65-18442

PRINTED IN THE UNITED STATES OF AMERICA

This book is dedicated to Mrs. Stanley McCormick because of her steadfast faith in scientific inquiry and her unswerving encouragement of human dignity.

Preface

The manuscript of this book was written and rewritten over a period of more than two years. During that period a break came in the apparent dam to publication on reproductive physiology and particularly its subdivisions concerned with reproductive behavior, conception, and contraception. The success of the oral contraceptives and the availability of many steroids of the types found effective have stimulated not only their experimental study but also numerous investigations in the general area of fertility control. What seemed at first to be a relatively uncomplicated task grew to rather formidable dimensions. To the experienced scientific writer this is evident from the need for over 1400 citations of experimental investigation. Even this does not tell the whole story, for in order to assess and select only the publications most pertinent to the subject matter of this book I have examined more than twice this number. Nevertheless, I have doubtless failed to cite a number of significant studies; certainly as the book is being processed and even as the faithful student reads it, accounts of new and relevant investigations are appearing. Nonetheless, I am confident that I have presented in this book the basic facts relative to the processes controlling fertility in higher animals. Moreover, I have attempted throughout to indicate the hiatuses in our knowledge, the questions demanding answers, and the probable needed directions of further research. To the inquiring mind this is perhaps not difficult, but the designation of meaningful areas for study requires also the familiarity of experience.

Indeed, it is because of a tolerably lengthy and fairly consistent experience that I have undertaken the writing of this book. As I have mentioned in the text much of the subject matter is taken directly from my work and that of my colleagues. Without the collaboration and stimulation of these colleagues even my most sanguine efforts would have been meager indeed. Their efforts are acknowledged following this preface.

A number of the donors mentioned in the acknowledgment have made possible a feature of our work not described in the text of this book. This is the travel to meetings and conferences and to laboratories, clinics, and other institutions concerned with aspects of the multifaceted discipline of reproductive physiology. As a result we have conferred and lectured in many countries of the world, seen at first hand the research needs and possibilities in almost every European, Asiatic, Central, and South American country. We have faced the hard fact of overpopulation in country after country, learned of the bleak demographic future, assessed the prospects for the practice of efficient fertility control. This has been a saddening and a heartening experience; saddening because of the sight of continuing poverty and misery, heartening because of the dedicated colleagues and workers seeking to overcome the handicap of excess fertility and to promote healthy reproductive function. Among these we have made many friends, found devoted students.

Perhaps most stimulating has been the recognition among these workers throughout the world of the need and merit of objective scientific study of all aspects of fertility and sterility. The ready acceptance of validated statistics, of experimentally substantiated facts, has encouraged our belief in the internationalism of scientific inquiry. Birth control and the allied areas of sexual physiology and sexual behavior have long been battlegrounds of opinion-voicers. They have suffered from clashes among differing culture patterns, theologies, moralities, even politics. These struggles still continue, but they are being more and more delimited by the findings of science. Objective appraisal is surely but slowly replacing heated partisanship.

It is the operation of the scientific process in the area of fertility control that this book attempts to portray. That process is neither the acme of efficiency nor the "Final Solver of All Problems." As is evident to all who read, it works by fits and starts, it leads to errors that must be painfully reviewed and critically rejected, it often dwells lengthily on minutiae, overstresses conditional findings, and for long periods fails to illumine factual obscurities. Nonetheless, it gets ahead, haltingly perhaps, but inevitably. The mystery and wonder of conception becomes describable in terms of gametes and their movements, in terms of fertilization reactions and the operation of replication mechanisms, in terms of oviduct chemistry and hormonal regulation. In each of these is also mystery and wonder, for there is still more to discover than we now know. But in the blazing or flickering light of what we do know a priori judgments and willful prejudices fade. And our considered and tested knowledge offers a firm basis for what we can and should do.

GREGORY PINCUS

Shrewsbury, Massachusetts
May, 1965

Acknowledgments

The list of my colleagues is a long one, beginning with my first research students at Harvard University, Drs. E. V. Enzmann and N. T. Werthessen, and continuing over a period of about thirty-five years to the present day. Reference to the work of most of these devoted research workers is made in the text, but I should like here to single out those who have long and consistently participated in my researches in reproductive physiology. Among them is Dr. M. C. Chang whose brilliant and illuminating animal experimentation is the product of an original mind which continues to stimulate all who talk and work with him, including myself. In this area of animal experimentation I have been particularly indebted for many years to the meticulous efforts of Miss Ann Merrill and Mr. T. Hopkins. In recent years Drs. E. S. E. Hafez, L. Fridhandler, E. B. Romanoff, M. X. Zarrow, T. Miyake, Y. Ogawa, N. Purshottam, B. Tamaoki, D. Layne, A. Erickson, Y. Kurogochi, A. Kulangara, G. Bialy, K. Arai, K. Yoshinaga, and U. K. Banik have contributed devoted and critical effort to investigations ranging from hormone assay and metabolism to pituitary-gonad relationships, to ovum and uterine biochemistry.

In the realm of advanced clinical investigation Dr. C. R. Garcia has been the skillful, knowledgeable, scientific physician dedicated to his patients as well as to the objectives of a far-ranging research effort. Working with him in our joint studies of human fertility control have been Drs. John Rock, E. Rice-Wray, M. Paniagua, A. Pendleton, F. Laraque, R. Nicolas, N. Borno, V. Pean, J. Shepard, E. E. Wallach, E. Klaiber, A. Parthenis, H. Rocamora, and J. Curet. The special studies in human subjects of the metabolism and biochemistry of hormones concerned with reproduction have occupied the skilled and thorough efforts of Mrs. L. P. Romanoff and her associates, of Drs. J. F. Tait, C. J. Meyer, D. S. Layne, and T. Golab. To all of these workers in the scientific vineyard and to their assistants and associates we express not only gratitude for devotion and unremitting effort but admiration for their enormous patient competence in ofttime difficult and always demanding research.

In addition to those associated immediately with my experimental studies there are many without whose efforts and cooperation neither this book nor the work which my colleagues and I have conducted would have been possible. Foremost among them is Elizabeth Pincus, my patient and beloved wife who has always been by my side through trying times, and who has sacrificed much to the forwarding of an effort in which she has had consistent faith. And to Dr. A. L. Raymond I am indebted not only for a staunch friendship but for the constant availability of his extraordinary critical acumen and scientific scepticism. Among his many colleagues at G. D. Searle and Company I have enjoyed particularly the chemical perspicacity of Drs. F. Colton, B. Riegel, and R. Burtner, the biological inventiveness and insight of Drs. F. J. Saunders, V. A. Drill, R. L. Elton, and R. A. Edgren, and the clinical knowledge of Drs. I. C. Winter, W. J. Crosson, W. Stewart, and G. R. Venning. Many other workers in the field of pharmaceuticals have been helpful with materials and advice. Their contributions have been acknowledged in our cited publications. So many men and women have aided us in our work that it would be difficult to name them all; they include workers at the Associacion pro Bienestar de los Familias in San Juan, Puerto Rico, social workers, nurses, and secretaries in Humacao, Puerto Rico, in Port-au-Prince, Haiti, at the Free Hospital for Women in Brookline, Massachusetts, and at the Worcester Foundation in Shrewsbury, Massachusetts. To my faithful and hardworking amanuenses, the Misses P. Purtell and J. Sanford I am especially indebted.

Finally I should here state my debt to those organizations and individuals that have made possible my work by grants-in-aid of research. Outstanding is G. D. Searle and Company and its officers who had the courage to assist my pioneer efforts when practically all other pharmaceutical companies had "cold feet." Other companies which have contributed to my work on reproduction are the Ciba Co., Julius Schmid, Inc., Merck, Sharp and Dohme Research Laboratories, Parke Davis and the Syntex Co. The Planned Parenthood Federation of America, the Population Council, the Josiah Macy, Jr. Foundation, and the Pathfinder Fund have made research grants for several aspects of our work. Most helpful have been Mrs. Albert D. Lasker, Mrs. James Faulkner, and Mr. Andre Meyer, each of whom have responded with generosity to special exigencies in our over-all efforts. The American Cancer Society has been the source of support for those phases of our work relating to tumorigenesis, cancer diagnosis, and control. And for thoughtful support of the training of research workers in reproductive physiology we have had a generous grant from the Ford Foundation.

Contents

I
Introduction

1. BACKGROUNDS

2. THE REPRODUCTIVE PROCESSES AND THEIR VULNERABILITIES IN MAMMALS

II
Animal Studies

3. SPERMATOGENESIS AND SEMEN

4. OVULATION

5. FERTILIZATION

6. FREE OVUM DEVELOPMENT

III

Clinical Studies

The Control of Fertility

I
INTRODUCTION

CHAPTER 1

Backgrounds

This book is primarily concerned with investigations into aspects of reproduction conducted by the author and his colleagues. It is, first of all, an attempt to summarize a collection of data hitherto either partially or not at all presented. Secondly, we shall attempt to indicate those avenues which hold promise for future investigation. Finally, we shall attempt an assessment of the implications of our understandings and ignorances.

Our own work began with a curiosity about mammalian fertilization and ovum maintenance (1). The evolution of internal fertilization and gestation in the oviducts has led to the establishment of various mechanisms for the safeguarding of the gametes and the conceptus. Because of their relative inaccessibility and certain difficulties in their maintenance *in vitro*, mammalian ova have, until lately, been used only to a limited extent as subjects for experimental study. Nonetheless, out of these early inquiries several findings emerged: (a) rabbit ova in moderately large number may be obtained by stimulating ovaries to superovulation by the administration of certain gonadotropic preparations (2)—this may be accomplished in a number of species of laboratory and domestic animals (3–5); (b) such ova may be readily fertilized (cf. 6), recovered, and cultured *in vitro*; (c) the fertilization of mammalian ova *in vitro* is accomplished with difficulty (7), and this may be due in large measure to the need for capacitation of the sperm, which is accomplished by their residence in the oviducts for a number of hours (8, 9); (d) fertilized rabbit eggs will readily

3

cleave at apparently normal rates *in vitro* (*1, 10*), but those of other species, e.g., guinea pig (*11*), rat (*12*), sheep, and goat (*13*), show only a limited amount of cleavage or none under a variety of culture conditions; (e) rabbit blastocyst growth under optimal conditions *in vitro* does not attain the rate observed *in vivo* (*14*) and growth *in vivo* is sharply limited by the action of ovarian hormones, particularly progesterone (*15, 16*); (f) energy for blastocyst growth *in vitro* appears to be derived from the Meyerhof glycolytic system provided enzyme maintenance by sulfhydril-containing compounds occurs (*17*), but probably special growth-promoting substances present in blood serum are additionally necessary.

In these probings into the range of mammalian egg activities extending from maturation and ovulation to implantation, several conclusions implied or stated have emerged as the basis for more recent investigations. First, the dependence of the ovarian follicle on pituitary gonadotropic hormones for stimulation to ovulation is emphasized. Second, fertilization is seen to be not merely a chance meeting of egg and sperm, but an event requiring maturation (capacitation) of sperm as well as eggs within the female reproductive tract. Third, the fertilized egg cleaves readily *in vivo* in the absence of ovarian hormones or even in the presence of an excess of estrogen (*18*), but unknown factors essential for normal cleavage are difficult to supply *in vitro*, at least for the eggs of certain species. Fourth, growth of the blastocyst in the uterus appears to depend upon a serum ultrafiltrate containing a variety of nutritional essentials and ordinarily made abundantly available as the result of progestational uterine states normally controlled by ovarian hormones, especially progesterone and possibly conditioned by some of its metabolites (*19*).

Each of these conclusions supports the possibility of control of fertility by manipulation of the ovum environment, and particularly its hormonal environment. Curiously, the cardinal basis for a large portion of the work forming the subject matter of this book was unapparent in these early researches. Thus we specifically found (and stated) that estrogen did not prevent ovulation in the rabbit (*18*), and, therefore, the important concept of a steroid feedback upon pituitary hormone production and/or release evaded us.

Actually, recent experimentation has indeed emphasized that many estrogens in otherwise "physiological" doses are poor or ineffective inhibitors of ovulation in the rabbit (20).

In 1937, Makepeace, Weinstein, and Friedman (21) noted the effectiveness of progesterone as an ovulation inhibitor in the rabbit, but the logical extension of this observation into a more intensive study of the nature of the progesterone action as well as the action of certain derivatives and putative metabolites were not reported by us until 1953 (22).

Why this "logical extension" occurred after a latent period of approximately 16 years is a question concerning which we have raised some speculation. Certainly, judging by publications, there was a period during which our own activities in this field fell to a minimum, both absolutely and relatively (Table 1). An examination

TABLE 1

PAPERS PUBLISHED BY THE AUTHOR AND NUMBERS LISTED BY AUSTIN (9) FOR
THE PERIOD 1934–1961

Period of publication	Total number of papers	Number concerned with reproduction and allied phenomena	Number in Austin's bibliography
1934–1937	29	18	35
1938–1941	35	22	34
1942–1945	26	12	18
1946–1949	27	5	70
1950–1953	54	10	119
1954–1957	60	21	150
1958–1961	41	27	132

of the bibliography of any book concerned with reproductive phenomena (e.g., 9) discloses similarly a minimum number of publications during the period 1942–1945, and a significant rise in output from 1950 on. In our own case, the special demands of "war" research accounted for a shift of interest to studies of adrenocortical function, particularly in relation to physical and mental stress, and this interest has continued to a greater or lesser degree. Indeed, World War II probably accounts for the lapse observed generally. In our case, the increase of activity as indicated by publications from 1950 on has been due to two overtly ascertainable factors:

(a) a visit from Mrs. Margaret Sanger in 1951 and (b) the emergence of the appreciation of the importance of the "population explosion."

At the time of her visit, Mrs. Sanger's interest in the world-wide dissemination of information on birth control was at high tide. Her experience as President of the International Planned Parenthood Federation had made her aware of the deficiencies of conventional contraceptive methods, particularly in underdeveloped areas of the world. Her hope, expressed to us, was that a relatively simple and fool-proof method might be developed through laboratory research. Drs. Chang and Pirie and I had already had some experience with hyaluronidase inhibitors in the rabbit (23) but we had found that such potent inhibitors could act only on direct contact with sperm and that there was no possibility of an effect by parenteral administration. Although some preliminary experiments by the late Dr. Abraham Stone had indicated that at least one of these inhibitors might be quite active as the component of an intravaginal preparation in the human, the limitations to its use still appeared to be rather formidable. Accordingly, Dr. Chang and I drew up a modest project proposal that received support under a grant from the Planned Parenthood Federation of America. Work under this grant resulted in the paper on the rabbits mentioned above (22) and in the finding that the compounds that we found to be potent as ovulation inhibitors in the rabbit were also quite active as antifertility agents in the rat (24).

The impetus to research, particularly on the physiology of reproduction, given by the recognition of the population explosion has been described a number of times (25, 26). Although the physiologist has generally been called upon to undertake research which might lead to easily effective and acceptable means of birth control, his role is indeed a much wider one. The modern-day investigator cannot be satisfied with the invention of a "cunning device." The present accumulated knowledge concerning reproductive processes indicates that the production of gametes, their transport and mating, their fusion, and the fate of the fertilized egg involves an intricate and delicately balanced set of sequential events. Interfering with this sequence at any of a large number of stages may have physiologic consequences that are not apparent on the surface. The research worker is therefore compellingly motivated to arrive at as complete an understanding as possible of the processes involved in the great act of reproduction. Furthermore, the understanding which the physiologist seeks must be imparted to others. Often both the nature and the degree of information that must be imparted for thorough understanding may be highly technical and even abtruse to professionals such as physicians in family planning clinics and public health workers.

Under the ivory tower conception of scientific research, much of the foregoing is irrelevant. More simply stated, the job of the scientist is to undertake experimentation and to publish the results of such experimentation. What happens thereafter is allegedly not his business. This concept has been dealt demoralizing blows, particularly during and since World War II. The rapid transition from the research laboratory to the world-wide application of significant discovery has demanded the attention of the scientist to two consequences of his activity. First of all, there is the need for training of fellow scientists, of students, of embryo research workers, of public health servants and so on. Willy-nilly the investigator has had to be also an educator. Secondly, chiefly because of the public alertness to scientific discovery, the research workers' talents have been invoked not only to help in making sure that the public is properly informed and not grossly misinformed, but also to consider questions of policy that are inevitably raised with the application of scientific discovery. Of course the outstanding present-day example of this is the role of the scientists concerned with the development of atomic energy. The physicists concerned with the development of atomic energy for eventual practical use have been cognizant of the wide implications of their discoveries and have often been eloquent about the proper use. In fact, the organization of the Federation of Atomic Scientists was instituted in large measure to ensure communication and debate concerning the uses and misuses of atomic energy.

Although in the opinion of many the population problem facing the community of men is as important as the problem of the development of atomic energy, the biological scientist has thus far not been vigorously communicative, nor is there indeed a Federation of Population Scientists. The economic and social aspects of the problem have indeed been expertly communicated by certain scientists concerned with demographic research. Their over- all statistical conclusions about the rate of increase of the human population, a number of their studies of specific national groups, their analyses of the effects of disease control have received wide attention in the public press, and the experts have produced publi- cations readily understandable by interested laymen (e.g., 27, 28). The physiological research worker thus far has for the most part confined his publication to scientific journals, and the publications by members of the medical profession (e.g., 29) have been chiefly concerned with medical practice in relation to birth control. The call-for-action programs (cf. 30) have largely passed over the re- search laboratory.

I suspect that the working physiologist is not too unhappy about being neglected by the "pointing-with-alarmers." It is not merely the residue of ivory-tower psychology that animates him. It is primarily his feeling that so much remains to be learned about the basic processes of reproduction, let alone practical control meas- ures. Nonetheless, we do have a formidable array of fact, and even some fairly tenable general principles. In an article designed to review the professional literature on the physiology of reproduction for the year June 1960 to June 1961 (31), I wrote an introductory paragraph which, I believe, epitomizes the problem facing a man attempting to assess the facts of our experimental science:

"Reproductive physiology is concerned with: (a) The genesis of the germ cells, (b) the factors involved in their maturation, safeguarding and release, (c) the mechanisms ensuring their trans- port and union, (d) the maintenance of embryogenesis and fetal life, (e) the delivery of young and the means of ensuring their immediate survival. Inquiry into the literature of these five appar- ently simple problems discloses a multiplicity of approaches, an extraordinary diversity of tangential data, the relevance of which to any central problem is often unjudgable, and an amassing of information so voluminous that its orderly classification requires computing machine techniques rather than the mind of a reviewer."

In this book we will not attempt to review all aspects of repro- ductive physiology. We shall be concerned with the experimental control of fertility as a specific biological problem.

REFERENCES

1. Pincus, G. 1936. "The Eggs of Mammals." Macmillan, New York.
2. Pincus, G. 1940. *Anat. Record* **77**, 1.
3. Smith, P. E., and Engle, E. T. 1927. *Am. J. Anat.* **40**, 159.
4. Robinson, J. T. 1950. *J. Agr. Sci.* **40**, 275.
5. Umbaugh, R. 1949. *Am. J. Vet. Res.* **10**, 295.
6. Adams, C. E. 1953. *In* "Mammalian Germ Cells" (G. E. W. Wolstenholme, ed.), p. 198. Little, Brown, Boston, Massachusetts.
7. Chang, M. C., and Pincus, G. 1951. *Physiol. Rev.* **31**, 1.
8. Chang, M. C. 1953. *In* "Mammalian Germ Cells" (G. E. W. Wolstenholme, ed.), p. 226. Little, Brown, Boston, Massachusetts.
9. Austin, C. R. 1961. "The Mammalian Egg." Charles C Thomas, Springfield, Illinois.
10. Gregory, P. W. 1930. *Contrib. Embryol., Carnegie Inst., Washington* **21**, 141.
11. Squier, A. H. 1932. *Contrib. Embryol., Carnegie Inst., Washington* **22**, 233.
12. Defrise, A. 1933. *Anat. Record* **57**, 239.
13. Winterberger, S., Danzier, L., and Thibault, C. 1953. *Compt. Rend. Soc. Biol.* **147**, 1971.
14. Pincus, G., and Werthessen, N. T. 1938. *J. Exptl. Zool.* **78**, 1.
15. Corner, G. W. 1928. *Am. J. Physiol.* **86**, 74.
16. Pincus, G., and Werthessen, N. T. 1937. *Am. J. Physiol.* **120**, 100.
17. Pincus, G. 1941. *Am. J. Physiol.* **133**, 412.
18. Pincus, G., and Kirsch, R. E. 1936. *Am. J. Physiol.* **115**, 219.
19. Pincus, G., and Werthessen, N. T. 1938. *Am. J. Physiol.* **124**, 484.
20. Pincus, G., and Merrill, A. P. 1961. *In* "Control of Ovulation" (C. W. Villee, ed.), p. 37. Pergamon Press, New York.
21. Makepeace, A. W., Weinstein, G. L., and Friedman, M. H. 1937. *Am. J. Physiol.* **119**, 512.
22. Pincus, G., and Chang, M. C. 1953. *Acta Physiol. Latinoam.* **3**, 177.
23. Pincus, G., Pirie, N. W., and Chang, M. C. 1948. *Arch. Biochem.* **19**, 388.
24. Slechta, R. G., Chang, M. C., and Pincus, G. 1954. *Fertility Sterility* **5**, 282.
25. Nelson, W. O. 1956. *Endocrinology* **59**, 140.
26. Pincus, G. 1959. *The Washington Post* (Aug. 2).
27. Hauser, P. M. 1960. "Population Perspectives." Rutgers Univ. Press, New Brunswick, New Jersey.
28. Fagley, R. M. 1960. "The Population Explosion and Christian Responsibility." Oxford Univ. Press, London and New York.
29. Guttmacher, A. F. 1959. "Babies by Choice or Chance." Doubleday, Garden City, New York.
30. Jones, J. M. 1962. "Does Overpopulation Mean Poverty?" Center for International Economic Growth, Washington, D. C.
31. Pincus, G. 1962. *Ann. Rev. Physiol.* **24**, 57.

CHAPTER 2

The Reproductive Processes and Their Vulnerabilities in Mammals

In this chapter we shall attempt to present a concise account of the sequence of processes essential to successful sexual reproduction in mammals. Presupposed is a sequence with basic features common to all mammals, and, couched in broad terms, this is indeed the case. A number of specialized, specific mechanisms, often fascinating in themselves, will be omitted, and, since we seek generalization, this chapter may appear elementary in content to some.

Processes in the Male

Beginning with the male we must consider the origin of spermatozoa, their maturation, and their discharge as fertilizing agents. The normal differentiation and growth of the testis in embryonic life is necessary for later fertility, and since the mammalian testis is not an independent, self-differentiating organ, factors controlling its development have been studied experimentally (32, 33). During certain critical stages (e.g., days 22 to 25 in the rabbit pregnancy) pituitary gonadotropic hormones act to stimulate normal testis differentiation. Among other endogenous agents,

10

the gonadal sex hormones and thyroid hormone may also affect fetal testis development. Sterilization by exogenous agents such as irradiation, cytotoxic substances, and other toxins is well known. A prenatal growth stimulus which may be followed by actual slight declines indicate that maternal gonadotropins are acting on the fetal testis (*34*).

In postnatal life there is a prepubertal period characterized by slow growth and minimal differentiation. This is illustrated in Fig. 1 and by data on rhesus monkey testis development (*35*).

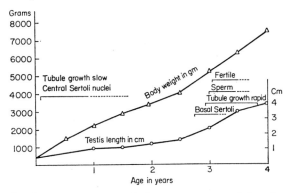

Fig. 1. Graphic representation of changes in testes of the rhesus monkey during development. Coordinates are body weight and age of animals, and length of testes. [From van Wagenen and Simpson (*35*).]

The prepubertal testis is clearly affected by anterior pituitary activity. This has been demonstrated by the arrest of its development and involution in hypophysectomized, immature males and its stimulation to accelerated growth by pituitary gonadotropin administration (*36*). Thus, any of several means of inhibiting gonadotropin action in immature animals will prevent the development of normal testis function. Actually, two pituitary hormones act upon the testis: (a) follicle-stimulating hormone (FSH) which stimulates testis growth and particularly spermatogenesis and (b) luteinizing (LH) or interstitial-cell stimulating hormone (ICSH) which primarily promotes male sex hormone secretion by the Leydig cells (cf. Fig. 2). The simultaneous administration of partially purified FSH and LH results in a synergistic stimulation of testis growth in hypophysectomized or immature rats (*37*). In rats hypophysectomized for 6 months. FSH produces some repair of spermatogenesis to the spermatid stage, and LH appears to act particularly on spermatocytes (38). The two administered together do not accomplish a complete restoration. Perhaps there is another factor essential for optimal spermatogenesis and present in the partially purified preparations of Greep *et al.* (37).

Actually, in the infantile male there is a period of "sterility" varying in length in different species from several days (in the rat) to many months (in primates) with rather mysterious origins. The testes appear to be refractory to pituitary hormones [although they may respond to other gonadotropins such as human chorionic gonadotropin (HCG)], there is generally an involution of the gonocytes prominent in fetal testes and the slow initiation of characteristic spermatogonial stem lines (34, 39, 40). The factors responsible for this natural postnatal involutional process are far from resolved. In the human male during the few days following birth the Leydig cells disappear and are replaced by undifferentiated, intertubular cells which remain as such for 10 or more years: until the initiation of puberty. The withdrawal of support by maternal HCG presumably accounts for the initial change, but what accounts for the persistence of inactivity? Are there intratesticular factors making for unresponsiveness to gonadotropins?

In Fig. 2 we present diagrammatically the reproductive organs of the mature male mammal. The basic processes essential to normal fertility are: (a) spermatogenesis in the testis tubules, (b) normal steroid secretion by the Leydig cells, (c) transfer of the sperm from the tubules to the epididymes, and (d) ejaculation of the sperm through the vasa efferentia, normally in a seminal fluid containing secretory products of the prostate and Cowper's glands and the seminal vesicles.

Spermatogenesis has numerous vulnerabilities. It is not an independent, self-sustaining process. The careful attention given in recent years to the progression of development from spermatogonia to spermatozoa has served to indicate rather exactly stages susceptible to fairly specific influence. In rats, 14 stages of development from spermatogonia to spermatozoa have been observable. In hypophysectomized rats development of spermatogonia to spermatocytes and of spermatocytes to spermatids (stage 7) occurs at a much reduced rate, but seven additional stages to mature sperm do not occur. Restoration to normal spermatogenesis is of course effected by proper gonadotropin administration. The developmental period and the length of time during which cryptorchid testes have been intra-abdominal condition the degree and nature of the damage to

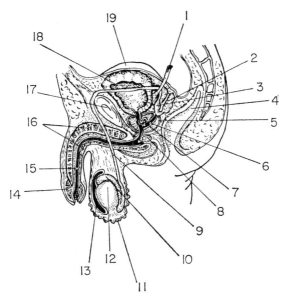

Fig. 2. Male genital organs shown in sagittal section.
1. Ureter; 2. Seminal Vesicle; 3. Ampulla; 4. Rectum; 5. Prostate; 6. Ejaculatory Duct; 7. Prostatic Utricle; 8. Cowper's Gland; 9. Ductus Deferens; 10. Epididymis; 11. Scrotum; 12. Testis; 13. Tunica Vaginalis; 14. Glans Penis; 15. Urethra; 16. Cavernous Bodies; 17. Pubis; 18. Urinary Bladder; 19. Peritoneum.

spermatogenetic stages. Nonetheless, complete loss of spermatogenetic potency will occur in long-term cryptorchidism with complete disappearance of spermatogenetic cells, even of Sertoli cells (41). Presumably the higher intra-abdominal temperature is immediately responsible for this germ-cell-line degeneration since Leydig cell involution is very much slower in cryptorchidism.

Other factors influencing spermatogenetic function have been discussed by Leathem (42). Fairly specific sensitivities to protein lack and to vitamins E, C, and biotin deficiency have been reported.

Less specific influences include thyroid excess, fat deficiency, and reduced intake of a number of vitamins. In later chapters we shall discuss the remarkable effects of steroids, some of which act upon spermatogenesis as inhibitors, others as stimulators, and others as both inhibitors and stimulators, depending upon the conditions.

There is no doubt that adequate steroidogenesis by testis interstitial tissue is essential for normal fertility. First of all sexual drive and normal copulatory function are clearly androgen-dependent. The fact that in some animals castration does not, under certain conditions, abolish copulatory behavior (43) does not detract from the finding that in practically all circumstances the androgen supply governs the frequency and intensity of such behavior (44) and that the development of sex patterns in man is androgen-dependent (45). Secondly, the maintenance of spermatogenesis appears to depend upon testis steroid. In 1934 Walsh, Cuyler, and McCullagh (46) made the arresting observation that spermatogenesis is maintained by testosterone administration to the hypophysectomized rat. This observation has been confirmed and extended to other species, and other steroids produced in the synthetic sequence leading to testosterone have also proven effective (34, 41). Thirdly, excessive steroid production by the testis may lead to sterility, presumably because the sex steroids in excess inhibit pituitary gonadotropin (47). Certainly excess exogenous steroid will be sterilizing, and estrogen has been found to be particularly effective in all mammals, including man (34, 48, 49).

The transfer of sperm from the tubules to the epididymides and their storage therein is, of course, essential to fertility. A number of factors are involved in the production of fertile epididymal sperm (50). Normal sperm transport and activity are androgen-conditioned. Movement into and along the epididymis appears to depend on muscular elements in the duct walls, the control of which is not too well understood (51). In the epididymis a maturation of the stored sperm occurs which is clearly androgen-dependent since castration sharply reduces the fertilizable life of epididymal sperm (52, 53) and androgen may restore it. The capacity for normal motility initiated in the testes is fully developed during sperm residence in the epididymis, but thus far none of the components of epididymal fluid taken alone or in various combination seems to be the responsible factor in this development (51). In the course of movement from head to tail, epididymal sperm develop not only capacity for motility but also for fertility (54). But despite some speculations on the role of the electrolytes in their environment no firm basis for the development change has been established.

Finally, the ejaculation of matured sperm in a seminal plasma having a number of specific properties is a step in the sequence of reproductive processes, the vulnerabilities of which have been scarcely probed. The number of spermatozoa needed in an ejaculate to assure fertility has been accurately determined in a number of species in which artificial insemination has been studied (51, 55, 56). Generally the limits are quite low and overproduction of sperm is often considered an atavistic anachronism. Nonetheless, variations in total count and in sperm concentration from species to species are enormous whereas the number of eggs ovulated tends to be rather small. Sperm count appears to depend chiefly on rates of spermatogenesis rather than on changes in the efferent ducts. Ejaculum sperm viability and fertility vary widely, depending on: (a) seminal plasma constitution and (b) sperm energetics and chemical constitution.

It is not possible to discuss here in detail the nature of seminal plasma and its role in normal fertilization. Since fertilization may be accomplished by insemination with epididymal sperm, seminal plasma has been considered unessential to normal fertilization. This does not mitigate against the fact that as a component of the ejaculate it does affect the sperm. It supplies a number of substances demonstrably utilized by sperm as sources of energy; indeed, it has been shown to enhance fertilizing capacity (57), and it may, in contrast, accumulate toxic substances from the blood, e.g., alcohol (58), sulfonamides (59). The possibility of differential secretion into prostatic or seminal vesicle fluid of highly potent spermicides is very much worth further study [cf. *145* (Ch. 3)]. The fascinating work of Mann and his associates on seminal fluid biochemistry (cf. *60*) merits amplification and advancement (cf. *61*).

Also we will not enter here into a detailed account of the biochemistry of ejaculate sperm. Thorough reviews have been published by Mann (*60*) and Bishop (*51*), among others. It suffices to point out here that ejaculate sperm have probably been the most studied organisms as vulnerable reproductive agents. Their susceptibilities to various lethal agents ranging from spermicidal antiseptics, to high temperature, to irradiation have been extensively explored. Exhaustive studies of their metabolism have been made, in part to determine if processes specific to sperm may offer a specific means of contraception. Thus far, the energy metabolism of mammalian sperm appears to devolve on oxidative and glycolytic systems found in mammalian tissues generally. The enzyme systems involved appear to be confined to the middle piece, and the sperm head acts principally as a rather inert bearer of the hereditary material. This suggests that mutagens may act on the head and most cell poisons on the middle piece, but probably at concentrations or under conditions no different from those used with other cells. What is suggested is that separating heads from middle pieces and tails may be quite valuable if it can be accomplished by simple, nontoxic means *in vivo*. Again the number of spermatozoa in an ejaculate may have a rather important bearing on the action of spermicides, antimetabolites, etc. As Chang (62) has pointed out, it is possible to reduce sperm count to $\frac{1}{100}$ or less and still have an adequacy of sperm for fertilization, and he has indeed observed almost normal fertility in the face of high intravaginal concentrations of several spermicides. Generally any agents inhibiting sperm motility must be close to 100% effective and irreversible in action (63).

Processes in the Female

A complex sequence of events essential to reproduction occur in the female mammal. For not only is there the necessity for the production, maturation, and discharge of ova, but also the need to ensure the meeting of sperm and ova, the proper delivery of the fertilized egg to its uterine couch, and the maintenance of the embryo and its safe delivery to the outside world.

Germ cell production in the female mammal is not analogous to spermatogenesis in the male. The primordial germ cells of the female embryo originate in the endoderm, migrate to the genital ridge, induce the formation of the fetal ovary and act as stem cells for the large crops of primordial ova present at birth. In spite of observations suggesting the cyclic formation of new germ cells from the germinal epithelium in sexually mature animals (*64, 65*) and the suggestion that such neogenesis is stimulated by estrogen (*66, 67*), recent studies suggest that the germinal epithelium is unessential for oogenesis in the adult mammal (*68, 69*). Postnatal oogenesis therefore involves the growth of primordial oocytes to adult size with concomitant development of their follicular adnexae. The end of the female's reproductive capacity comes when the neonatal crop of oocytes is entirely depleted. Accompanying the growth of ova and follicles are atretic processes which may halt development at any stage. Ordinarily the ovum reaches mature size in relatively immature follicles (Fig. 3). Although a functional ovum ripening

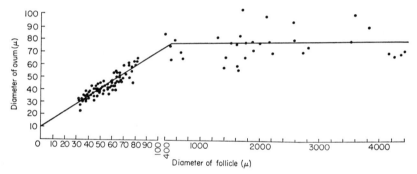

Fig. 3. Regression lines relating size of ovum to follicle size in human ovaries. [From Green and Zuckerman (*69a*).]

may occur, the growth of follicles to preovulatory sizes appears necessary only for the attainment of capacity to ovulate and then to form corpora lutea. What stimulates some primordial ova to grow and leaves others unstimulated? Presumably all immature oocytes are potentially stimulable, but no experimental procedure has pinpointed the responsible stimulators. Indeed, hypophysectomy does not appear to affect noticeably the primordial oocytes and their follicular cells [cf. *1* (Ch. 1), 69]. Responses to gonadotropin are obvious only in follicles containing full size ova and generally on the verge of or just initiating antrum formation. In prepubertal monkeys, FSH administration may stimulate new follicle formation and particularly the growth of small follicles, but no new ova are formed (70, 71). Thus many possible vulnerabilities of primordial and growing oocytes remain to be determined. It is, of course, well known that irradiation will completely destroy all oocytes, leaving a sterile ovary capable of estrogen secretion (72). More subtle inhibitors or stimulators of oogenesis remain to be found.

Figure 4 is a diagrammatic representation of the adult female mammal's reproductive tract. The growth and development of antrum-containing follicles, pre-ovulatory swelling, and follicle rupture are ovarian processes under pituitary control. They do not

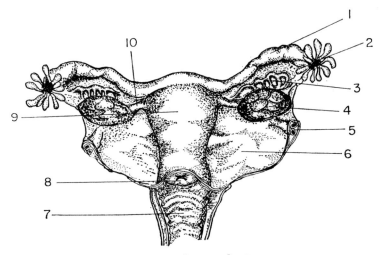

FIG. 4. The female reproductive tract.
1. Uterine Tube; 2. Ostium Abdominale; 3. Epoöphoron; 4. Ovary; 5. Ovarian Vessels; 6. Broad Ligament; 7. Vagina; 8. External Cervical Os; 9. Uterus; 10. Ovarian Ligament.

occur in hypophysectomized animals and may be reinitiated by proper replacement with pituitary gonadotropins. It is fairly well established that FSH is the hormone that stimulates follicle growth and that it synergizes with LH in inducing pre-ovulatory swelling and ovulation (37). Thus any interruption of the pituitary-gonad relationship will lead to sterility due to the failure of ovulation. Actually, pituitary secretion of FSH and LH and particularly their accurately phased secretion rates are in turn controlled by a hypothalamic neurohumoral activity. Specific hypothalamic centers appear to be concerned with the stimulation of FSH secretion, others with LH secretion, still others with the inhibition of LH secretion; these centers in turn are affected by circulating ovarian steroid and steroid hormone metabolites (*73, 74*). A complex of vulnerabilities is immediately apparent. Many of them have received intensive experimental study to be described in later chapters.

The ovary, like the testis, performs a dual function: It produces germ cells (and the apparatus needed for their eventual ovulation) and secretes steroid hormones. Normal ovarian steroidogenesis is also dependent on pituitary gonadotropins. Although the steroidogenic sequences in ovarian tissue have been characterized in some detail, the exact role of pituitary gonadotropins remains to be determined. The major precursor of ovarian hormones is cholesterol and the reactions leading to the hormonal steroids are presented in Fig. 5. The major secretory products of the ovary are the estrogens, estradiol and estrone, and progesterone. Androgen, probably as androstenedione, is also secreted in limited amount. Abnormal steroidogenesis by the ovary generally means a sterile ovary, e.g., in the Stein-Leventhal syndrome or in ovaries with arrhenoblastoma (*75, 76*). Qualitative or quantitative variations in ovarian steroid secretion will have definite effects on pituitary gonadotropin secretion. Thus excess estrogen inhibits FSH synthesis and liberation in practically all animals studied. Its effect on pituitary LH may vary (depending on species, age, quantity, and time in sex cycles) from suppression to stimulation. Moreover, estrogen interacts with progesterone in effects on LH release. Progesterone, in properly timed administration at relatively low dose, may stimulate ovulation in a number of animals (*36*) and women (*77*). At higher doses, however, and normally during the luteal phase of the female sex cycles, progesterone acts as an inhibitor of LH release, and thus of ovulation [*20, 22* (Ch. 1), *36*].

The ovulating follicle heals after rupture and forms the corpus luteum which is the primary ovarian tissue of pregnancy since it secretes progesterone in amounts adequate to maintain gestation. Before the corpus luteum is formed for full function, ova are fertilized. Fertilization may be affected by corpus luteum function

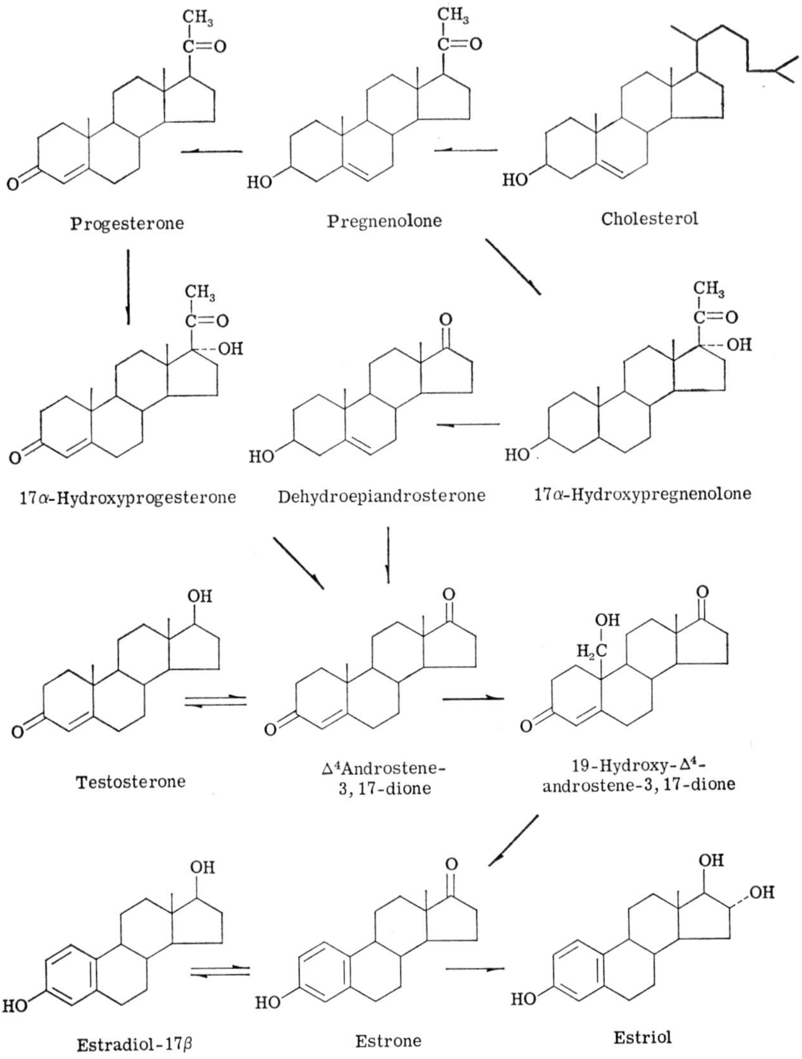

Progesterone   Pregnenolone   Cholesterol

17α-Hydroxyprogesterone   Dehydroepiandrosterone   17α-Hydroxypregnenolone

Testosterone   Δ⁴Androstene-3, 17-dione   19-Hydroxy-Δ⁴-androstene-3, 17-dione

Estradiol-17β   Estrone   Estriol

FIG. 5. Pathways of estrogen biosynthesis.

since it has been shown that progesterone administration may inhibit fertilization (78), perhaps by its effects on uterine and tubal motility, or, more probably, by its action on sperm-fertilizing capacity (*vide infra*). Anything which acts to prevent normal corpus luteum function will act as an infertility agent. Since the corpus luteum is supported by a pituitary tropic hormone (LTH) the upsetting of the normal pituitary-ovary relationship will affect processes supported by corpus luteum secretions. Thus estrogens may inhibit LTH secretion in some species (36, 79). LTH has been found to be identical with prolactin in test animals, but though it is produced during human pregnancy its concentration is low, especially in early months, its functional activity dubious, and no effective activity of administered prolactin has been demonstrated. Corpus luteum maintenance and progesterone secretion by the placenta in the human appear to be under the control of placentally secreted human chorionic gonadotropin (HCG) (80, 81).

Even with an adequately maintained normally active corpus luteum, the hazards to successful early pregnancy are considerable. Fertilization may be accomplished only if properly capacitated sperm (*vide* Chapter 5, p. 89) reach the oviducts during the relatively brief period when the discharged ova are capable of fertilization. Sperm capacitation in the uterus is inhibited in the luteal phase and by progesterone administration (82). Ovum potency for fertilization may be as brief as 5 hours, as in the hamster (83), somewhat longer than 30 hours in the ferret (84), and in the human appears to be no less than 6 and no longer than 24 hours (85). The transport of sperm through the uterus and into the Fallopian tubes has been the subject of much investigation. Correlations between the type of uterine and tubal contraction and the rates of sperm passage have been sought for a number of species (cf. 51 and 86). Estrogen and progestin each have characteristic effects on oviduct muscular contraction, and their absence or presence in excess clearly affect the concentration of sperm in various parts of the tract. For rapid sperm transport, a third hormone, oxytocin, appears to be essential, at least in certain species, due to its action on uterine motility (87, 51). Ovarian steroid hormone-oxytocin interrelationships have been studied intensively, particularly in relation to parturition (88), but fertility control by them as a complex governing sperm movement merits detailed inquiry.

Once the egg has been successfully fertilized it passes through two significant stages before it implants into the uterine wall: (a) a period of tubal passage during which cleavage occurs and (b) a period of intrauterine passage during which development and growth as a blastocyst supervenes.

Although the rate of cleavage appears to be exempt from the influence of endogenous regulatory factors, the rate of passage through the Fallopian tubes is not. Thus, estrogen may act to prevent exit into the uterus (by "tube-locking" the ova) and progesterone hastens the passage of ova into the uterus (89). Since cleaving ova are actively dividing, antimitotic agents should have a suppressive or even a lethal effect. We shall see later that certain agents do act directly on tubal ova in experimental animals, perhaps by antimitotic action (90).

The period of blastocyst development has been found to be labile to many agents. We have indicated in Chapter 1 (p. 4) that such lability is due to: (a) a progestin-controlled uterine environment and (b) dependence on specific nutritive factors. We have shown in addition that a glycolytic activity in rabbit ova is first seen in the late morula and early blastocyst stages (91). Thus, in the blastocyst, both oxidative and glycolytic systems are available for attack. Furthermore, the rabbit blastocyst behaves metabolically exactly like tumor tissue in exhibiting the Pasteur reaction shift (92). Thus a variety of antitumor agents should act as inhibitors of blastocyst development, and there is some experimental evidence for this (93).

In addition to agents acting directly on the uterine ova, substances or conditions affecting normal hormonal action upon the uterus will affect fertility. Normally estrogen and progesterone act synergistically upon the uterine endometrium to prepare it for nidation, although progesterone alone may accomplish this [19 (Ch. 1)]. An upset of hormonal balance essential to progestational proliferation may be accomplished by excess of estrogens or by other antiprogestins (94, 95), or perhaps by anti-estrogens, or even by an excess of progesterone (96). A number of years ago we presented data that certain phenanthrene derivatives administered to rabbits might act to inhibit the endometrium-stimulating capacity of progesterone without affecting its blastocyst growth-stimulating action, whereas others affected ovum but not endometrial growth (97). The basis for such antagonisms is far from evident. Although a number of alterations in endometrial metabolism are progestin-conditioned, their relationship to pregnancy maintenance may be incidental. Thus the remarkable stimulation of endometrial carbonic anhydrase by progestin administration to the rabbit is not seen in the rat, and indeed is reversed in the mouse (i.e., progesterone reduces uterine carbonic anhydrase activity). Does this imply a nonessential role of carbonic anhydrase to implantation? The endometrium prepared for nidation exhibits changes in concentrations of various enzymes, vitamins, lipids, etc. Ovarian hormones affect processes varying from histamine release to cholesterol synthesis. Even the susceptibility of the uterus to infection is exaggerated in the luteal phase of the cycle probably by reducing the rate of leucocyte infiltration (98, 99).

The processes affecting blastocyst development and endometrial proliferation appear to reach a culmination at or shortly after the time of implantation. Thus, in the rabbit the uterine concentrations of carbonic anhydrase, ascorbic acid, histaminase, adenosine triphosphate, alkaline phosphatase, and so on reach a maximum at about the sixth day of pregnancy and within one or more days show a decline in concentration (100). Agents which reduce the levels of these endometrial constituents (e.g., estrogens and other antiprogestins) prevent implantation, although whether this is by virtue of specific action on one or more of these constituents is unknown. Implantation may be prevented by direct lethal action on blastocysts of various antimetabolites (101). Similarly, the implanted embryos are susceptible to abortion by upsets in hormonal balance, by direct toxic actions of antimetabolites and by compounds inducing abnormal uterine contraction (93, 101, 102).

In the foregoing account of various vulnerabilities of male and female reproductive processes, no attempt has been made at a comprehensive description of the numerous susceptible stages in the intricate sequences leading to the production of viable young. Some eight years ago, Nelson made just such a summing up [25 (Ch. 1), 103], and a conference devoted chiefly to the subject was held in 1959 (*104*). It is abundantly evident that upsettable, delicately balanced mechanisms operate at practically every step. What happens when disruption is attempted? Indeed, what kind of attempts at disruption have been made? What are the overall consequences of such attempts? These are the questions we propose answering in the chapters concerned with the experimental control of fertility. Initially we shall describe experimental studies with animals. Later we will examine meaningful clinical applications of the animal studies. If our attention appears to be concentrated on what amounts to antifertility studies, this is because they are in fact most numerous. But it should never be forgotten that experimental sterility studies are pertinent to problems of naturally occurring sterility. The large number of infertile couples (commonly said to number 10% of all marriages) are living examples of the vulnerabilities of reproductive processes. Indeed, when one considers all of the hazards involved, the production of viable young may often appear to be a minor miracle.

REFERENCES

32. Jost A. 1953. *Recent Progr. in Hormone Res.* **8**, 397.
33. Burns, R. K. 1961. *In* "Sex and Internal Secretions" (W. C. Young, ed.), Vol. I, p. 76. Williams & Wilkins, Baltimore, Maryland.
34. Albert, A. 1961. *In* "Sex and Internal Secretions" (W. C. Young, ed.), Vol. 1, p. 305. Williams & Wilkins, Baltimore, Maryland.
35. Van Wagenen, G., and Simpson, M. E. 1954. *Anat. Record* **118**, 231.
36. Greep, R. O. 1961. *In* "Sex and Internal Secretions" (W. C. Young, ed.), p. 240. Williams & Wilkins, Baltimore, Maryland.
37. Greep, R. O., Fevold, H. L., and Hisaw, F. L. 1936. *Anat. Record* **65**, 261.
38. Lostroh, A. J. 1963. *Acta Endocrinol.* **43**, 592.
39. Clermont, Y., and Perey, B. 1957. *Am. J. Anat.* **100**, 241.
40. Daoust, R., and Clermont, Y. 1955. *Am. J. Anat.* **96**, 255.
41. Nelson, W. O. 1937. *Cold Spring Harbor Symposia Quant. Biol.* **5**, 123.
42. Leathem, J. H. 1961. *In* "Sex and Internal Secretions" (W. C. Young, ed.), Vol. I, p. 666. Williams & Wilkins, Baltimore, Maryland.
43. Beach, F. A. 1961. "Hormones and Behavior." Harper (Hoeber), New York.
44. Young, W. C. 1957. *In* "Hormones, Brain Function and Behavior" (H. Hoagland, ed.), p. 75. Academic Press, New York.
45. Money, J. W. 1961. *In* "Sex and Internal Secretions" (W. C. Young, ed.), Vol. II, p. 1383. Williams & Wilkins, Baltimore, Maryland.

46. Walsh, E. L., Cuyler, W. K., and McCullagh, D. R. 1934. *Am. J. Physiol.* **107**, 508.
47. Venning, E. H. 1942. *Rev. Can. Biol.* **1**, 571.
48. Heckel, N. J., and Steinmetz, C. R. 1941. *J. Urol.* **46**, 319.
49. de la Balze, F. A., Mancini, R. E., Bur, G. E., and Irazu, J. 1954. *Fertility Sterility* **5**, 421.
50. Risley, P. L. 1963. *In* "Mechanisms Concerned with Conception" (C. G. Hartman, ed.), p. 73. Macmillan, New York.
51. Bishop, D. W. 1961. *In* "Sex and Internal Secretions" (W. C. Young, ed.), Vol. II, p. 707. Williams & Wilkins, Baltimore, Maryland.
52. Moore, C. R. 1928. *J. Exptl. Zool.* **50**, 455.
53. Young, W. C. 1929. *J. Morphol.* **47**, 479.
54. Young, W. C. 1931. *J. Exptl. Biol.* **8**, 151.
55. Walton, A. 1958. *J. Roy. Agr. Soc. Engl.* **119**, 63.
56. Farris, E. J. 1950. "Human Fertility Problems of the Male." The Author's Press, White Plains, New York.
57. Chang, M. C. 1949. *Proc. Soc. Exptl. Biol. Med.* **70**, 32.
58. Farrell, J. I. 1938. *J. Urol.* **40**, 62.
59. Osenkoop, R. S., and MacLeod, J. 1947. *J. Urol.* **58**, 80.
60. Mann, T. 1954. "The Biochemistry of Semen." Wiley, New York.
61. White, I. G., and MacLeod, J. 1963. *In* "Mechanisms Concerned with Conception" (C. G. Hartman, ed.), p. 135. Macmillan, New York.
62. Chang M. C. 1960. *Fertility Sterility* **11**, 109.
63. Bishop D. W. 1962. *Physiol. Rev.* **42**, 1.
64. Allen, E. 1923. *Am. J. Anat.* **31**, 439.
65. Evans, H. M., and Swezy, O. 1931. *Mem. Univ. California* **9**, 119.
66. Stein, K., and Allen, E. 1942. *Anat. Record* **82**, 11.
67. Bullough, W. S. 1946. *Phil. Trans. Roy. Soc.* **B231**, 453.
68. Enders, A. C. 1960. *Anat. Record* **136**, 491.
69. Zuckerman, S. 1962. "The Ovary." Academic Press, New York.
69a. Green, S. H., and Zuckerman, S. 1951. *J. Anat.* **85**, 373.
70. Simpson, M. E., and Van Wagenen, G. 1953. *Anat. Record* **115**, 370.
71. Simpson, M. E., and Van Wagenen, G. 1958. *Fertility Sterility* **9**, 386.
72. Brambell, F. W. R., Parkes, A. S., and Fielding, V. 1927. *Proc. Roy. Soc.* **B101**, 95.
73. Villee, C. A., ed. 1961. "The Control of Ovulation." Pergamon Press, New York.
74. Rothchild, I. 1962. *Fertility Sterility* **13**, 246.
75. Parkes, A. S. 1950. *Rec. Progr. Hormone Res.* **5**, 101.
76. Warren, J. C., and Salhanick, H. A. 1961. *J. Clin. Endocrinol. Metab.* **21**, 1218.
77. Rothchild, I., and Koh, N. K. 1951. *J. Clin. Endocrinol.* **11**, 789.
78. Boyarsky, L. H., Baylies, H., Casida, L. E., and Meyer, R. K. 1947. *Endocrinology* **41**, 312.
79. Austin, C. R., and Bruce, H. M. 1956. *J. Endocrinol.* **13**, 376.

80. Browne, J. S. L., Henry, J. S., and Venning, E. H. 1938. *J. Clin. Invest.* **17**, 503.
81. Zarrow, M. X. 1961. *In* "Sex and Internal Secretions" (W. C. Young, ed.), Vol. II, p. 958. Williams & Wilkins, Baltimore, Maryland.
82. Chang, M. C. 1958. *Endocrinology* **63**, 619.
83. Chang, M. C., and Fernandez-Cano, L. 1958. *Anat. Record* **132**, 307.
84. Hammond, J., and Walton, A. 1934. *J. Exptl. Biol.* **11**, 307.
85. Hartman, C. G. 1936. "The Time of Ovulation in Woman." Williams & Wilkins, Baltimore, Maryland.
86. Hartman, C. G. 1939. *In* "Sex and Internal Secretions" (C. H. Danforth and E. A. Doisy, eds.), p. 630. Williams & Wilkins, Baltimore, Maryland.
87. Van Denmark, N. L., and Moeller, A. N. 1951. *Am. J. Physiol.* **165**, 674.
88. Caldeyro-Barcia. R., and Heller, H. (eds.) "Oxytocin." Pergamon Press, New York.
89. Blandau, R. J. 1961. *In* "Sex and Internal Secretions" (W. C. Young, ed.), Vol. II, p. 797. Williams & Wilkins, Baltimore, Maryland.
90. Segal, S. J., and Nelson, W. O. 1958. *Proc. Soc. Exptl. Med.* **98**, 431.
91. Fridhandler, L., Hafez, E. S. E., and Pincus, G. 1957. *Exptl. Cell Res.* **13**, 132.
92. Fridhandler, L. 1961. *Exptl. Cell. Res.* **22**, 303.
93. Jackson, H. 1959. *Pharmacol. Rev.* **11**, 135.
94. Alden, R. H. 1942. *J. Exptl. Zool.* **90**, 159.
95. Pincus, G., and Merrill, A. P. 1963. *In* "Perspectives in Biology" (C. F. Cori, V. G. Foglia, L. F. Leloir, and S. Ochoa, eds.), p. 56. Elsevier Press, New York.
96. Cochrane, R. L., and Meyer, R. K. 1954. *Proc. Soc. Exptl. Biol. Med.* **86**, 705.
97. Pincus, G., and Werthessen, N. T. 1938. *Proc. Roy. Soc.* **B126**, 330.
98. Casida, L. E. 1953. *In* "Mammalian Germ Cells" (G. E. W. Wolstenholme, ed.), p. 262. Little, Brown, Boston, Massachusetts.
99. Heap, R. B., Robinson, D. W., and Lamming, G. E. 1962. *J. Endocrinol.* **23**, 351.
100. Delgado, R., and Fridhandler, L. 1964. *Exptl. Cell Res.* **34**, 45.
101. Adams, C. E., Hay, M. F., and Lutwak-Mann, C. 1961. *J. Embryol. Exptl. Morphol.* **9**, 468.
102. Thiersch, J. B. 1959. *Proc. 6th Intern. Congr. Planned Parenthood, New Delhi, India,* p. 157.
103. Nelson, W. O. 1956. *Acta Endocrinol. Suppl.* **28**, 7.
104. Hartman, C. G. (ed.). 1963. "Mechanisms Concerned with Conception." Macmillan, New York.

II
ANIMAL STUDIES

CHAPTER 3

Spermatogenesis and Semen

In the preceding chapter we indicated the spermatogenic processes susceptible to experimental alteration. In general there have been two approaches to the inhibition of spermatogenesis. The first is an attack on the pituitary-testis axis. The second is an attempt to inhibit directly any or all spermatogenic stages.

Pituitary and Gonadotropin Inhibition

Generally the attack on the pituitary-testis axis has involved steroid administration to test animals. The most powerful steroid inhibitors of spermatogenesis are the estrogens. They presumably act by inhibiting FSH production and release. In immature animals, testicular descent may be prevented as well as spermatogenesis (105) and this effect is observed with the use of either natural or synthetic estrogen (106). Compounds derived from plants, e.g., genistein (107) or synthetics such as methylbisdehydrodoisynolic acid (108) or hydroxypropriophenone (109) all appear to inhibit pituitary gonadotropin. Despite some indication of species differences, practically all experimental animals thus far studied have shown quite similar responses. Although spermatogenesis is clearly estrogen-labile, Leydig cell function also may be inhibited [34 (Ch. 2), 110]. Thus both FSH and LH activity are affected by estrogen (111). Accompanying the reduction of seminiferous tissue to spermatocytes, spermatogonia, and Sertoli cells and the atrophy of Leydig cells, there is often a hyalinization of the basement mem-

29

brane. Mating reactions in males so treated tend to be abolished. Restoration of normal sexual behavior in male rats made sterile by estrogen injections (dienestrol diacetate, 20 μg twice a week) was accomplished by a single intratesticular implant of testosterone (3 mg). As long as the implant remained, normal behavior persisted in the face of continued estrogen (112).

"The varied effects obtained by injecting male hormone into normal and hypophysectomized rats depend upon the nature of the androgen, the dose, the length of the treatment period, and the age of the animals when treatment is begun." With this statement, Albert [34 (Ch. 2)] introduces his detailed account of the effects of androgenic steroid on testis function. We have already noted that androgen will maintain spermatogenesis in the hypophysectomized animal; this activity in a variety of steroids appeared to be very nearly inversely proportional to their androgenicity (113). In rats with intact pituitaries following relatively low doses (e.g., 100 μg testosterone propionate per day or less), spermatogenesis is suppressed, presumably due to pituitary gonadotropin inhibition in the face of inadequate androgen for direct seminiferous epithelium support [34 (Ch. 2), 114]. At practically all doses used, and in all species studied, Leydig cell atrophy occurs. Therefore, androgen, like estrogen, inhibits both FSH and LH, but here because of its endogenous biological activities this tends to be obscured in male recipients. Androgen also has the property of reducing the atrophying effects of estrogen (110, 115), presumably because of its supportive effect on testis tubules. The suppressive action of testosterone may be potentiated by simultaneous administration of molybdenum (116). Other steroids have been generally less studied, chiefly because of minimal or ill-defined effects. Thus cortisol and related steroids appear to have at most minor depressive effects on testis weight in young rats, but not in older test animals [34 (Ch. 2), 117]. In man, large doses of cortisone given for rheumatoid arthritis do not affect the histological appearance of the testes (118). Deoxycorticosterone in large doses over long periods of time to rats arrests testis growth and may even cause Leydig cell atrophy. This may be due to pituitary inhibition for it has no effects on the testes of adrenalectomized rats (119).

The investigation of effects of progestins on spermatogenesis in experimental animals have been quite limited, and indeed have been antedated by studies in man. Recently we have examined a series of progestins and related compounds. Pertinent data of these studies (*120*) are presented in Table 2.

Here it will be seen that a standard estrogen causes marked inhibition of testis growth, complete suppression of spermatogenesis, Leydig cell atrophy, and pituitary hypertrophy at doses at which a standard androgen causes moderate growth inhibition, no, or some inhibition of spermatogenesis, no significant effect on Leydig cells or pituitary weight (Expt. 1). Progesterone, at the dosage employed, had no discernible effect, whereas two very weak 19-norprogestational compounds did inhibit testis growth and spermatogenesis with minor or no effects on Leydig cells and the pituitaries (Expt. 2). A third weak progestin which is also a fairly active androgen is a powerful inhibitor of testis growth, completely suppresses spermatogenesis and causes moderate Leydig cell atrophy with no effect on pituitary weight (Expt. 3). Two additional 19-norsteroids of moderate progestational potency (Expts. 4 and 5) significantly inhibit testis growth, partially inhibit spermatogenesis with no or slight effect on Leydig cells, and one but not the other tends to stimulate pituitary growth. In contrast, a highly active synthetic progestin (Expt. 6) at low dose significantly stimulated testis and pituitary weight, and at higher dose had little or no significant effects. The estradiol effect is closely mimicked by an impeded estrogen (Expt. 5) except that pituitary weight is unaffected by it.

Included in Table 2 also are some experiments with several androgen derivatives having varied androgenic-anabolic properties. Among them, one 19-norsteroid (Expt. 9) is extremely active as an inhibitor of testis growth and spermatogenesis, but has no significant effect on pituitary size. One compound, a very active protein anabolic agent, has exhibited rather paradoxical effects. By injection at modest dose (5 mg) it clearly inhibits testis growth and spermatogenesis; at five times this dose testis growth is still inhibited, but significantly less than at the lower dose and spermatogenesis is normal (Expt. 7). This same substance administered orally has no inhibitory effects at all, and at moderate dose appears to increase testes growth and pituitary weight (Expt. 8). For the

TABLE 2

The Effect of Various Steroids on Testis Weight, Spermatogenesis, Leydig Cell Appearance, and Pituitary Weight of Juvenile Rats[a]

Experiment no. and compound administered	Total dose (mg)	Testis weight (mg/gm body weight)	Spermatogenesis	Leydig cells	Pituitary weight (mg/gm body weight)
Experiment 1					
Control	—	10.7 ± 0.20	Normal	Normal	0.041 ± 0.001
Estradiol-17β	0.4	3.7 ± 0.27[b]	Complete suppression	Atrophic	0.056 ± 0.001
Estradiol-17β	1.0	3.8 ± 0.28	—	—	0.054 ± 0.004
Estradiol-17β	2.0	2.6 ± 0.21	Complete suppression	Atrophic	0.071 ± 0.007
Testosterone	0.4	9.4 ± 0.40	Normal	Normal	0.040 ± 0.001
Testosterone	1.0	8.9 ± 0.27	—	—	0.041 ± 0.002
Testosterone	2.0	8.6 ± 0.38	Inhibited	Normal (?)	0.038 ± 0.004
Experiment 2					
Control	—	10.6 ± 0.60	Normal	Normal	0.045 ± 0.002
Progesterone	2.0	10.5 ± 0.13	Normal	Normal	0.047 ± 0.003
17α-Ethynyl-19-nor-Δ^{3,5}-androstadiene-3,17-diol diacetate	1.0	7.0 ± 0.74	Inhibition	Almost normal	0.054 ± 0.002
	5.0	4.6 ± 0.68	Inhibition	Slight atrophy	0.048 ± 0.001
17α-Ethynyl-Δ$^{5(10)}$-estrene-3,17-diol	2.0	9.2 ± 0.66	Normal	Normal	0.046 ± 0.003
17α-Ethynyl-Δ$^{5(10)}$-estrene-3,17-diol	10	8.1 ± 0.89	Partial inhibition	Normal	0.060 ± 0.002
Experiment 3					
Control	—	11.2 ± 0.11	Normal	Normal	0.044 ± 0.004
17α-Vinyl-19-nortestosterone	2.0	5.4 ± 0.86	Complete suppression	Moderate atrophy	0.039 ± 0.005
17α-Vinyl-19-nortestosterone	10	3.5 ± 0.24	Complete suppression	Moderate atrophy	0.037 ± 0.001

Experiment 4					
Control	—	10.9 ± 0.38	Normal	Normal	0.042 ± 0.001
17α-Ethyl-19-nor-Δ⁴-androstene-3,17-diol-3-propionate	2.0	8.4 ± 0.68	Normal	Normal	0.040 ± 0.001
	10	6.4 ± 0.45	Partial inhibition	Normal	0.046 ± 0.003
Experiment 5					
Control	—	11.0 ± 0.79	Normal	Normal	0.050 ± 0.001
17α-Ethinethinyl-19-nor-Δ³,⁵-androstadiene-3,17-diol diacetate	2.0	9.9 ± 0.77	Normal	Normal	0.059 ± 0.003
	10	7.8 ± 0.41	Partial inhibition	Slight atrophy	0.058 ± 0.001
Δ¹,³,⁵-Estratriene-2,3,17-triol triacetate	0.2	6.1 ± 0.53	Complete suppression	Atrophic	0.048 ± 0.001
Experiment 6					
Control	—	10.6 ± 0.37	Normal	Normal	0.045 ± 0.003
6-Keto-17-acetoxyprogesterone	2.0	12.5 ± 0.68	Normal	Normal	0.055 ± 0.001
6-Keto-17-acetoxyprogesterone	10	10.8 ± 0.11	Normal	Slight atrophy	0.048 ± 0.001
Experiment 7					
Control	—	11.1 ± 0.38	Normal	Normal	0.039 ± 0.002
19-Nor-Δ⁴-androstene-3,17-diol diproprionate	1.0	10.5 ± 0.60	Normal	Normal	0.041 ± 0.001
19-Nor-Δ⁴-androstene-3,17-diol diproprionate	5.0	4.8 ± 0.44	Inhibition	Slight atrophy	0.036 ± 0.001
19-Nor-Δ⁴-androstene-3,17-diol diproprionate	25	7.2 ± 0.44	Normal	Slight atrophy	0.036 ± 0.001
Experiment 8					
Control	—	10.4 ± 0.58	Normal	Normal	0.041 ± 0.001
19-Nor-Δ⁴-androstene-3,17-diol diproprionate[c]	1.0	11.3 ± 0.34	Normal	Normal	0.041 ± 0.001
19-Nor-Δ⁴-androstene-3,17-diol diproprionate[c]	5.0	14.4 ± 0.67	Normal	Normal	0.045 ± 0.001
19-Nor-Δ⁴-androstene-3,17-diol diproprionate[c]	25	11.2 ± 0.28	Normal	Normal	0.044 ± 0.002

(Continued)

TABLE 2 (*Continued*)

Experiment no. and compound administered	Total dose (mg)	Testis weight (mg/gm body weight)	Spermatogenesis	Leydig cells	Pituitary weight (mg/gm body weight)
Experiment 9					
Control	—	10.8 ± 0.48	Normal	Normal	0.047 ± 0.001
4-Chloro-17α-methyl-19-nortestosterone	1.3	4.1 ± 0.51	Complete suppression	Moderate atrophy	0.048 ± 0.001
4-Chloro-17α-methyl-19-nortestosterone	6.6	3.7 ± 0.60	Complete suppression	Moderate atrophy	0.050 ± 0.001
Experiment 10					
Control	—	10.4 ± 0.31	Normal	Normal	0.040 ± 0.002
6α-Methyl-17α-ethynyl-Δ4-androstene-3β,17β-diol	1.0	10.1 ± 0.53	Normal	Normal	0.040 ± 0.005
	5.0	10.8 ± 0.28	Normal	Normal	0.040 ± 0.003
6α-Methyl-17α-ethynyl-Δ4-androstene-3β,17β-diol	25	10.2 ± 0.43	Normal	Normal	0.043 ± 0.003
Experiment 11					
Control	—	11.5 ± 0.76	Normal	Normal	0.049 ± 0.001
11β-Hydroxy-Δ4-androstene-3,17-dione	2.0	11.8 ± 0.53	More sperm	Normal	0.052 ± 0.003
11β-Hydroxy-Δ4-androstene-3,17-dione	10	12.0 ± 0.33	More sperm	Normal	0.052 ± 0.001
Experiment 12					
Control	—	10.4 ± 0.20	Normal	Normal	0.041 ± 0.001
1,2-Epoxyandrostane-3,17-dione	2.0	10.5 ± 0.29	Normal	Normal	0.043 ± 0.001
1,2-Epoxyandrostane-3,17-dione	10	10.9 ± 0.30	Normal	Normal	0.044 ± 0.001

[a] Twenty-six-day-old male rats received single daily injections for 3 weeks. Testicular biopsies were taken weekly. Autopsy was conducted 24 hours after the last injection.

[b] *Underlined* values significantly different from control values.

[c] Administered by gavage.

two other compounds listed, no inhibitory action is demonstrated; indeed one, a typical adrenal androgen, seems to stimulate sperm production (Expt. 11).

Kincl *et al.* (*121*) also have reported high antigonadotropic activity in males for the 19-norsteroid of Expt. 9 as well as for 2α-methyl-17β-hydroxyandrostan-3-one. They also found two 19-methylated androgen derivatives (2α-fluoro-17α-ethynyltestosterone and 2-benzoyloxymethylene-17α-methyl-17β-hydroxyandrostan-3-one) to be quite active. The compound of Expt. 3 and its 17α-ethynyl analog have been found antigonadotropic in male rats, and the effect is neutralized by either FSH or LH administration. Other progestins, related to 17-acetoxyprogesterone, were reportedly inactive (*122*), but Merkle (*129*) has found that 17-acetoxyprogesterone, its 19-noranalog and several 17-substituted 19-norsteroids produce in mature rats a 50% reduction in Leydig cell volume after 2 weeks injection of 1 mg per day. 17α-Ethynyl-19-nortestosterone causes tubule and Leydig cell atrophy in rabbits (*123*). Testicular atrophy, particularly tubular, has been reported to occur in mice receiving nidroxyzone (*124*).

In castrate rats the 19-norsteroids, methyl-, ethyl-, and ethynyl-19-nortestosterone as well as norethynodrel inhibit castration changes in the anterior pituitary, e.g., the increase in basophils and the appearance of "signet-ring" cells (*125*). Androgenic activity of 17-methyl- and 17-ethynyl-19-nortestosterone and of 17-acetoxy-6-methylprogesterone has been observed in castrated guinea pigs (*127*). Evidence that the antigonadotropic effect of androgenic steroids is mediated by the hypothalamus has been presented by Davidson and Sawyer (*126*).

A number of nonsteroidal substances act as inhibitors of spermatogenesis by affecting pituitary gonadotropin secretion. Among these may be listed: (a) an extract of *Polygonum hydropiper* (L.), active in male mice (*128*), (b) 2-amino-5-nitrothiazole (Enheptin), active in the male fowl but not in the rat (*130–132*), (c) 1α-methylallylthiocarbamoyl-2-methylthiocarbamoylhydrazine which is active in rats, dogs, and monkeys, but not in mice, guinea pigs, rabbits, or horses (*133*).

Sterility in the male induced by a number of experimental procedures has been attributed to effects on the pituitary-testis relationship. Thus Meschaks (134) has described an aspermatogenesis occurring in bulls transported for long distances. The condition is characterized by symptoms of adrenocortical hyperactivity. Similarly, hyperadrenocorticism accompanies the sterility occurring when experimental animals are taken to high altitude; indeed, there is some evidence that an "abnormal" adrenocorticosteroid is secreted (135). An alarm reaction may also underlie the sterility induced in rats by auditory seizures (136).

Direct Effects on Testis Tissue

Many compounds which appear to act directly on the seminiferous tissue have been studied in experimental animals. Their classification is rather difficult because their chemical natures are quite diverse. Nonetheless, we may subdivide them as follows: (a) substances causing irreversible testis damage, (b) nitrofuranes and compounds having similar effects, (c) mitosis inhibitors, (d) cytotoxic, alkylating agents, (e) antimetabolites, and (f) antibodies.

Examples of irreversibly damaging agents are cadmium salts and erucic acid. The former, when administered to male rats, causes destruction of the seminiferous tubules with varying damage to the Leydig cells (137). Doses effective by parenteral administration may cause other toxic symptoms, but intratesticular injection at low dose is quite effective and systemic effects are avoided (138, 139). Intratesticular injection of cadmium chloride in the monkey results in total destruction of the seminiferous epithelium and temporary Leydig cell atrophy (140). Scrotal inunction in rats has similar effects (141). The sterilizing action in rats may be due to induced vascular ischemia rather than a direct action on the tubule cells (142). Animals in which cadmium chloride has no antispermatogenic effect include the grass frog, the pigeon, the rooster, the armadillo, and the opossum (143). Erucic acid fed to rats has similarly destroyed spermatogenetic tissue, but left the interstitial tissue intact (144). Kamboj and Kar (145) have recently observed testis tubule and Leydig cell degeneration following intratesticular injection of 35 salts of metals and rare earths. Nine of their compounds were also active on subcutaneous injection.

Furacin, furadroxyl, and furadantin, originally reported as testis cytotoxins (*146*), the nitrofuranes, have been studied extensively by Nelson and colleagues [*103* (Ch. 2), *147*], and examined as to their effects on carbohydrate metabolism in the testis (*148*). All three compounds are active in rats when given by mouth and arrest spermatogenesis at the pachytene stage in primary spermatocytes (*149*). This effect takes several weeks to be fully evident, presumably because of the length of residual postmeiotic stages. There appears to be no effect on Leydig cells and toxicity is low. Recovery of normal spermatogenesis occurs following withdrawal of the drugs and the rate of recovery is improved by steroid administration (*149*). As a drug with similar or reversible effects on spermatogenesis, Jackson [*93* (Ch. 2)] mentions 5-chloro-2-acetylthiophene. More recently certain antimalarial drugs have been found to be nitrofurane-like in their action on the testis (*150*). That these bis(dichloroacetyl)diamines do not act via the pituitary has been rather clearly demonstrated by administering them to hypophysectomized rats in which spermatogenesis has been maintained by testosterone proprionate (TP) injection. Their characteristic effect on spermatogenetic tissue is seen, but no alteration of the accessory organ response to the TP (*151*). Their effectiveness is seen in dogs and monkeys as well as rats (*152*). Most recently certain dinitropyrroles have effectively sterilized rats by single dose administration once every 4 weeks; spermatogenesis is halted at the spermatocyte stage and recovers when treatment is withdrawn (*153*). These compounds are active in guinea pigs and rabbits as well as rats (*154*) and apparently inhibit spermatogenesis stimulation by gonadotropin (*155*). Normal Leydig cells and accessory organs indicate absence of effect on processes concerned with androgenesis (*156*). Certain toxic effects seen in dogs have discouraged much further study (*156*).

Colchicine and trimethylcolchicinic acid methyl ether are antimitotic agents which have been tested in males. The former has inhibited spermatogenesis in rabbits with no apparent effect on Leydig cells (*157*). The latter has proven less toxic and has shown clear mitosis inhibition of mouse spermatogonia (*158*, *159*).

The observations of testicular lesions caused by aliphatic nitrogen mustards administered to mice (*160*) have led to a number of investigations with these and other cytotoxic agents [reviewed most recently by Jackson (161)]. In rats the ethyleneimines as well as the nitrogen mustards prevent the later stages of spermatogenesis and full recovery occurs some weeks after discontinuance (162–164). In a careful quantitative study, Steinberger (165) finds triethylenemelamine to have a rather specific effect on Type A spermatogonia in rats. This compound fed to starlings at low dose (0.1 mg per day) causes testis regression (166). A rather unique effect of ethyleneimino compounds in the rat is upon epididymal sperm which are rendered infertile. The sulfonoxy alkanes, of which Myleran is an outstanding example, have also received rather careful study as reversible sterilizing agents in the male rat (167–169). Lethal action on spermatozoa and late spermatids was obtained with methyl-methanesulfonate and ethylmethanesulfonate. Isopropylmethanesulfonate interfered with spermatogonia and spermatocytes and had a longer latent period to sterility. Thus by varying the dose administered and the type of sulfonate both the latent period to sterility and the duration of the sterile period could be determined. Activity was seen after oral as well as parenteral administration. Similar data have been obtained for rabbits (170) and mice (161). A special sensitivity of embryo rat gonads to busulfan has been reported (171).

Ova fertilized by sperm of male rats partially sterilized by Myleran show abnormal cleavage and only a few implant and develop normally (161). Preimplantation deaths of mouse zygotes developing from ova fertilized by sperm from heavy water (30% D_2O) ingestors have been reported (172). Male rabbits treated with thalidomide have exhibited numerous sterile matings and deleterious effects on some of the viable progeny (173).

Antimetabolites have been studied chiefly in the female, but ethionine, a methionine analog, damages the seminiferous epithelium of test rats (174). It does not affect the pituitary and its effect is completely inhibited by the simultaneous administration of methionine (175). Among other antimetabolites, 6-azauracil riboside has been found to inhibit mitosis and spermatid transformation to spermatozoa (176). Among a number of antibiotics, Chloromycetin proved to be a remarkable inhibitor of oxygen

uptake, lactic acid production, and motility of dog spermatozoa
(177); its effect in vivo is not known.

The possibility of producing antibodies to sperm has been
extensively explored in experimental animals. Excellent reviews of
this subject have been made by Segal (178) and Tyler (179).
Table 3, adapted from Tyler's review, demonstrates that immunity
against both heterologous and homologous sperm may be induced,
that spermatogenesis may be suppressed in guinea pigs and rats
by immunization with testicular extracts combined with adjuvant,
and that fertility may be impaired in various experimental animals
by immunization with testicular or seminal materials. Among the
many problems raised by these immunization procedures, the following deserve more than passing attention: (a) the presence of
anti-antibodies; (b) the feeling that anaphylactic reactions may be
more easily induced than antifertility effects; and (c) the difficulties in developing practical isoimmunity procedures (cf. 180).
Edwards (181), reviewing these difficulties, hopes that acrosome
autoantigens may be sufficiently active to induce significant immunity to sperm. McLaren (182) has reported a long-lasting
reduction of fertility in female mice which received live mouse
sperm intraperitoneally three times a week for 7 weeks. Among
the young produced no abnormalities were seen. Some special antigenic effect of live sperm may be involved.

A significant alteration in male fertility in certain mammals may
be had by changing the scrotal, and, therefore, the testis temperature. Increasing this temperature by various devices, e.g., wrapping
testes in insulating material (183), heating with infrared lamps
(184) or with microwaves from a radar source (185), has led to
spermatogenesis inhibition entirely similar to that seen in experimental cryptorchidism. Rats, mice, rams, dogs, guinea pigs, and
monkeys (186, 187) have all shown this reversible heat-induced
depression of spermatogenesis. In the rat, heating the testes specifically affects premeiotic division of primary spermatocytes and
spermatids in step 1 of spermiogenesis (188). A single exposure
may have effects lasting some weeks. Local application of cold to
the guinea pig scrotum also results in testicular degeneration (189).
Interestingly, such cold treatment in rabbits will induce disintegra-

TABLE 3

EXPERIMENTS OF IMMUNIZATION OF VARIOUS ANIMALS WITH TESTICULAR OR SEMINAL MATERIALS[a]

Key to abbreviations: Fe− = impaired fertility; Fe+ = normal fertility; Sp− = aspermatogenesis; Sp± = impaired spermatogenesis; Sp+ = normal spermatogenesis; Ag = agglutination; An = anaphylaxis; C-F = complement fixation; Im = immobilization; Ly = lysis; Pr = precipitation; Pr-D = agar diffusion; Pr-E = immunoelectrophoresis; Pr-F = fluorescent antibody.

Immunizing antigen	Immunized animal	Type of reaction or of effect	Investigators[b]
1. Human, bull, and guinea pig semen	Guinea pig	Im	Metchnikoff (1899)
2. Human semen; dog and bull semen or testis emulsions	♀ Rabbit	Pr	Farnum (1901a, b)
3. Human, bull, stallion, boar, and ram spermatozoa	Rabbit	Pr	Schütze (1902)
4. Human semen and testis extracts	Rabbit	Pr	Strube (1902)
5. Human spermatozoa	Rabbit	Pr	Uhlenhuth (1904)
6. Human spermatozoa	Guinea pig	An	Minet & Leclerc (1911)
7. Human spermatozoa	Guinea pig	An	Verger (1911)
8. Human, bull, dog, rabbit, guinea pig seminal fluid, or testis extract	Rabbit	Antiserum toxic to male guinea-pigs	Gräfenberg & Thies (1912)
9. Human spermatozoa	♀ Rabbit	Fe+ (in rabbits), Ag, Im	Dittler (1920)
10. Human spermatozoa	Rabbit	Pr	Dervieux (1921, 1923)
11. Human, boar, bull, stallion semen, sperm extracts or seminal fluids	Rabbit	Pr (species and semen specific)	Hektoen (1922); Hektoen and Manly (1923); Hektoen and Rukstinat (1928)
12. Human or rat spermatozoa	♀ Rat	Fe−, Ag, Im	McCartney (1923a, b)
	♂ Rat	Sp−	McCartney (1923a, b)
	Pregnant rat	Abortion	McCartney (1923a, b)
13. Human semen	Woman, vaginally	No serol. reactions of serum with semen	Bodnar & Kamniker (1925)

14. Human sperm	Woman	C-F, Im	Rosenfeld (1926)
15. Human, bull, ram, rabbit, guinea pig, and rat spermatozoa	Rabbit	Ag, Im, change in electrophoresis of spermatozoa	Mudd (1927); Mudd & Mudd (1929)
16. Human and rat testis and epididymis brei	Rat	Ag, inhib. of Graafian follicles	Morimune (1931)
17. Human and other spermatozoa (50° to 100°C)	Woman, ♀ rat	Fe−, Im, Pr	Baskin, (1932 1935, 1937)
18. Human sperm extract	Woman	Fe−, Im (cervical secretion)	Escuder (1936)
19. Human and rat spermatozoa	Woman	Fe−, Ag, Im	Rodriquez-Lopez (1936)
20. Human, bull, ram, rat, mouse spermatozoa	♀ Rabbit, ♀ Rat	C-F, Im	Henle (1937, 1938)
21. Human, bull, dog, rabbit, guinea pig sperm heads and tails	Rabbit	Ag, C-F (head- and tail-specific antibodies)	Henle et al. (1938)
22. Human seminal plasma	Rabbit	Pr	Ross (1946)
23. Human semen, washed spermatozoa, or heads and tails	Rabbit	Ag	Kibrick et al. (1952a, b)
24. Human sperm head lipoprotein; also bull, boar, ram, dog	Rabbit	Ag	Dallam & Thomas (1953)
25. Human spermatozoa	Rabbit	Ag	Bocci & Notarbartolo di Villarosa (1956)
26. Human, boar, and rabbit spermatozoa	Rabbit	Fe+ (rabbit), Ag, Im, Ly, Pr	Matsuura (1956)
27. Human and rabbit semen and epididymal or testicular spermatozoa	Rabbit and guinea pig	Ag, C-F, Pr-D (not sperm specific)	Weil (1960); Weil & Finkler (1958, 1959); Weil & Rodenburg (1960); Weil et al. (1956, 1959)
28. Human serum	Horse	Pr-E with human seminal plasma	Hermann et al. (1958a, b); Hermann (1959)

TABLE 3 (*Continued*)

Immunizing antigen	Immunized animal	Type of reaction or of effect	Investigators[b]
29. Human and buffalo semen	Rabbit	Pr-D	Rao & Sadri (1959, 1960)
30. Monkey spermatozoa	Rabbit	C-F	Bruck (1907)
31. Rabbit testis and epididymal brei	Guinea pig	Ag, Im	Metchnikoff (1900)
32. Rabbit and guinea pig spermatozoa	Rabbit	Fe− (passive immun. of ♂ mouse), Ly	London (1902a, b)
33. Rabbit and guinea pig spermatozoa	♀ Rabbit and ♀ guinea pig homologously	Fe−, Ag, An, C-F, Im	Savini & Savini-Castano (1911a, b)
34. Rabbit and guinea pig testes or spermatozoa	Rabbit	Im	Metalnikoff & Strelnikoff (1913)
35. Rabbit testes	♀ Rabbit	Fe−	Venema (1916)
36. Rabbit spermatozoa	♀ Rabbit	Fe−, Ag, Im	Dittler (1920)
37. Rabbit spermatozoa	Same rabbit	Im	Guyer (1921, 1922)
38. Rabbit spermatozoa	Domestic fowl	Fe− (in ♂ rabbits), Sp−, Ag, Im, Ly	Guyer (1921, 1922)
39. Rabbit spermatozoa or testis extract, rat spermatozoa	♀ Rabbit	Fe−, Im	Pommerenke (1928)
40. Rabbit spermatozoa	♀ Rabbit	Fe−, Ag, C-F, Im	Ardelt (1931, 1933)
41. Rabbit testis implants	♀ Rabbit	Fe−	Motta (1932)
42. Rabbit, rat, bull, ram, and guinea pig spermatozoa	Rabbit, rat, also vaginally	Fe+ by active im., Fe+ by passive im., Fe− by mixing spermatozoa and anti-serum, C-F, Pr	Parsons & Hyde (1940)
43. Rabbit, dog, goat, and bull semen; rabbit, goat, guinea pig, rat, and mouse epididymal spermatozoa	Rabbit, goat, and sheep	Ag, Pr (flocculation)	Smith (1949a, b)

44. Rabbit semen	Heifer	Fe− (spermatozoa mixed with antiserum)	Kiddy et al. (1959)
45. Rabbit semen + Adj. rabbit, see 8, 15, 21, 26, 27, 63, 66, 76, 77, 81, 85	Rabbit	Ag, C-F, Im, Pr-D	Edwards (1960b)
46. Guinea pig testis and epididymal brei	Rabbit, guinea pig	Im	Metalnikoff (1900, 1910)
47. Guinea pig testis	Guinea pig	Im	Adler (1909)
48. Guinea pig testis brei	♂ Guinea pig	C-F, Im (autologous and isologous spermatozoa)	Fitzgerald (1910)
49. Guinea pig spermatozoa	♂ and ♀ guinea pig	Fe−, Sp−, Im	Kennedy (1924)
50. Guinea pig semen	♀ Guinea pig	Fe−	Castoro (1926)
51. Guinea pig or bull spermatozoa, guinea pig testis extract	♀ Guinea pig	Fe+	Henle et al. (1940)
52. Guinea pig testis homog. + Adj.	♂ Guinea pig	Sp−	Voisin et al. (1951, 1958); Voisin and Delaunay (1955)
53. Guinea pig testis extracts + Adj.	♂ Guinea pig	Sp−, C-F, Im	Freund et al. (1953)
54. Guinea pig sperm head and tail extracts, sem. plasma	Rabbit	Pr-D, Pr-E	Pernot (1956)
55. Guinea pig spermatozoa + Adj.	Guinea pig	Sp−, C-F	Narpozzi (1957)
56. Guinea pig spermatozoa or testis homog. + Adj.	♂ and ♀ guinea pig	Fe−, Sp−, C-F	Katsh (1957, 1958a, b, c, 1959a); Katsh & Bishop (1958)
57. Guinea pig spermatozoa or testis extract	Guinea pig	Pr-F	Baum (1959)
58. Guinea pig testis homogenate + Adj.	♀ Guinea pig	Fe−, Ag, An, Pr	Isojima et al. (1959)
59. Guinea pig spermatozoa or testis homog. + Adj.	Rabbit and ♂ and ♀ guinea pig	Ag, Pr-D	Isojima & Stepus (1959)
60. Guinea pig testes guinea pig, see 1, 8, 15, 21, 32, 34, 35, 42, 43, 63, 66, 77, 90	♂ Guinea pig	Sp−	Waksman (1959)

the rabbit and the antigonadotropic assays in rats and mice may be explicable on the ground that the former measure LH effects. Alternatively, there may be marked species differences in sensitivity to estrogens and progestins, with rats and mice being primarily estrogen-sensitive and rabbits being more progestin-labile. Or a combination of both possibilities may apply. In baboons ingesting 17-acetoxyprogesterone for several months, a normal pituitary cytology is seen *pari passu* with ovarian follicle atrophy, corpus luteum and stroma shrinkage (255).

Unfortunately no direct comparisons between species of the mode of action of antigonadotropins have been expressly made. Assay of pituitary and serum LH in estrogen-treated rats suggests inhibited synthesis by estrogen (256). The urinary excretion of gonadotropin in castrated female rats has been inhibited by the administration of progesterone, testosterone, the cyclopentyl enol ethers of progesterone, and 17α-acetoxyprogesterone and the n-octylenolic ether of dihydrotestosterone (257). This appears to be a specific block of gonadotropin since other pituitary hormones are unaffected, at least by progesterone (258). However, in these experiments no distinction has been made between FSH and LH, so whether a differential effect is exerted by these compounds remains to be seen.

Antigonadotropins and the Hypothalamus

In general, the remarkable antigonadotropic potency of estrogens in rats and mice has been attributed to their inhibition of FSH synthesis and/or release rather than to LH inhibition. The prevention of ovulation *in vivo* actually requires rather high estrogen dosage, although ovarian growth is inhibited at quite low dose. Certainly evidence for an estrogen-sensitive anterior hypothalamic center has been repeatedly offered (220, 259). Thus in the rabbit estrogen implants into the posterior median eminence of the hypothalamus initially block copulation-induced ovulation and later lead to ovarian atrophy (260, 261). In rats this area appears to be the basal tuberal median eminence which is also androgen sensitive (262). Nonetheless, evidence has been presented indicating that in the rat two hypothalamic centers may be concerned

with LH release, one which controls the continuous release of LH
and which is not estrogen sensitive, and another involved with the
cyclic release of LH essential for ovulation (263). Bogdanove
(264) has observed that the pituitary castration cells of female rats
will regress in the region of ovarian or estrogen implants whereas
estrogen pellet implants into the hypothalamus are less effective,
dose for dose. He believes, therefore, that the hypothalamus is an
area from which estrogen is distributed to the pituitary via the
hypothalamic pituitary portal system.

A quite specific hypothalamic extract of bovine or rat tissue
which acts on direct injection into the rat pituitary (265) demonstrates the possibility of a specific LH-releasing stimulator. This
direct acting luteinizing hormone releasing factor (LHRF) has
been extracted from the median eminence of the sheep hypothalamus; its administration to rats on day 3 of diestrus or day 7 of
pseudopregnancy leads to ovulation which, of course, never occurs
normally at these times (266). A hypothalamic center for the production of a specific LHRF is indicated by: (a) the activity of
acid extracts of hypothalamus but not of similar extracts of brain
and cerebellum (267); (b) the ovulation-inducing potency of purified sheep hypothalamic extracts in rats made anovulatory by hypothalamic lesions and the inefficacy of vasopressin and oxytocin
in such animals (268); and (c) the isolation of a low molecular
weight polypeptide from beef stalk median eminence extracts
active in rats (269). The existence of this hypothalamic center has,
of course, been the subject of much experimental probing since
the finding that ventral anterior hypothalamic lesions in rats which
lead to persistent vaginal cornification (270) are followed also by
ovarian atrophy (271). A number of hypothalamic lesion studies in
rats thereafter obviated certain areas as LHRF sources (272–274).
Using the plasma LH of the estrogen-progestin treated ovariectomized female rat as an index of LHRF action, McCann and
co-workers (275, 276) have found activity primarily in median
eminence extracts. They have demonstrated absence of activity in
cerebral cortex extracts and activity in only pharmacological
amounts of vasopressin and epinephrine. The full identification of
LHRF now found by two groups (276, 277) to be heat-stable with

a molecular weight of less than 3000 should do much to simplify experimental studies in this important area.

A center concerned with the inhibition of LH release has also been suggested (277, 278). In addition Nalbandov (279) presents evidence supporting the hypothesis that LH release leading to ovulation must be preceded by a withdrawal of FSH stimulation. There may be, therefore, several hypothalamic centers involved in a series of closely integrated events essential to the release of ovulating hormone. The relative lability of each of these centers to various hormonal steroids may underlie a number of the thus far unexplainable phenomena of potency variations, both inter- and intraspecific. It has been observed that cortisol acetate crystals implanted in the rabbit anterobasal hypothalamus only inhibit stress-induced pituitary ACTH release (280). This then is the region for ACTH blockage by corticosteroids. Nonetheless, progesterone is a weak ACTH-blocking agent in rats and 6-methyl-17-acetoxy-progesterone is as active as cortisol (281). Such ramifications of synthetic steroid actions in the CNS have scarcely been explored. When we consider also the evidence for a steroid-sensitive mating center in the brain (282), specifically localized in the posterior and central medial basal hypothalamus in the rabbit (283), the complex of interrelationships is further emphasized. Indeed, studies of amygdala lesions (284, 285) and stimulation (286) suggest a fairly specific nervous pathway to the LH-releasing center.

As indicated above, most of the studies on hypothalamopituitary interrelationships have been concerned with LH-controlling mechanisms. Detailed studies of FSH-controlling factors have been meager indeed. Although lesion experiments in several species suggest an FSH-releasing center (272) no preparation comparable to LHRF has been made. The alleged special sensitivity of FSH secretion in the rat to estrogen has been challenged (287). Inhibition of follicle ripening in rats by lynestrenol and absence of such inhibition but clear ovulation blocking by its 6α-methyl derivative (288) suggests that the former may bind to an FSH-releasing center, the latter to an LH-releasing center. Studies of the localization of radioactive steroids in brain tissues seem requisite even if localization is not entirely indicative of functional activity.

Although there appears to be no question of the presence of specific steroid-sensitive hypothalamic centers for the neurohumoral control of gonadotropin release, some question has been raised as to a direct effect of steroids on the anterior hypophyseal gonadotropic cells. We have already cited experiments on the effects of estrogen pellet implants in rat pituitaries (264). McCann and Ramirez (276) find such implants much less effective than hypothalamic implants. Since complete blockage of endogenous LH release requires both estrogen and progesterone in the ovariectomized rat an effect (perhaps contributed by progesterone) on pituitary tissue may be involved. In a study of the aldehyde fuchsin-negative basophile cells of the castrate rabbit receiving estrogen pellet implants, Kanematsu and Sawyer (289) found a small reduction (from 5.3 to 3.7%) in hypophysis-implanted tissues, a somewhat greater reduction (to 2.9%) with anterior median eminence implantation, but a marked reduction (to 0.7%) with posterior median eminence basal tuberal region implants.

Just what biochemical events occur in steroid-sensitive hypothalamic areas under various conditions is practically completely unknown. Choline acetylase activity, particularly in the posterior hypothalamus of the rat, increases markedly after castration, tends to be low at estrus, and is reduced in castrates by estrogen administration (290). Progesterone has no effect and testosterone tends to increase this activity (291). A cholinergic mechanism responsive to estrogen is suggested.

Although we are far from having an explanation of the ovulation-inhibiting and antigonadotropic action of a variety of steroids, practically every month evidence is published for new and often highly effective substances. Thus 4-hydroxylation of certain moderately active steroids enhances antigonadotropic potency in some and abolishes it in others (292); halogenation of the 17α-ethynyl sidechain of several steroids has increased activity (293); the acetophenone derivative of 16α, 17α-dihydroxyprogesterone is a potent antifertility agent in the female rat but not in the male rat (294, 295); alkylation at carbon 6 and further unsaturation in ring B has produced promising ovulation inhibitors (296, 297). Among the 13β-substituted gonanes produced by total synthesis, the 13-methyl derivative is most active as an antigonadotropin, but least active as a progestin (298). Methylation at carbon 7 of 19-nortestosterone markedly increases its antifertility and uterotropic properties (299); certain retrosteroids show similar actions (300).

Inhibition of Exogenous Gonadotropin

We have indicated that ovulation inhibition by steroidal agents fundamentally appears to involve interference with hypothalamic processes governing pituitary gonadotropin synthesis and release. The possibility of direct action of steroidal agents upon the ovarian follicle has received little experimental support, but some evidence of such direct action may be found in the literature. Thus Bradbury (301) has demonstrated a growth-stimulating action of estrogen injected directly into the immature rat ovary, accompanied by corpus luteum formation and an increased responsivity to exogenous gonadotropin. Aron *et al.* (302) have observed this same increased sensitivity to gonadotropin in adult rats with intra-ovarian estrogen injections. Holmes and Mandl (303) accept the evidence of the lack of effect of norethynodrel upon ovaries in hypophysectomized rats and the ready responsiveness to exogenous gonadotropin of the ovaries of norethynodrel-treated rats (304, 305) as evidence of pituitary inhibition as the source of norethynodrel action. Nonetheless, they find some indication for a direct inhibitory action of this compound upon ovarian follicles. Actually, inhibition *in vitro* by estrogen of gonadotropin-induced ovulation in frog ovaries has been reported (306), but comparable data for mammals are either lacking or somewhat difficult to interpret (cf. 307 studies of follicles grown in tissue culture). A variety of compounds have been administered by Kar *et al.* (308) to immature rats responding to exogenous gonadotropin. Of eight compounds found to inhibit the ovarian weight response, chloroacetocatecheol was the most active and 2,3,5-trimethyl hydroquinone next; 4-methyl uracil and vanillin increased uterine weight and inhibited ovarian weight increase, and vanillin was not only the most uterotropic but also inhibited the induced ovulation. An estrogen-like effect of these latter compounds is suggested.

We have studied the effects of various compounds, including steroids, upon gonadotropin-induced ovulation in immature mice

TABLE 11

The Effects of Various Compounds on Quantified Ovulation

Compound	No. animals in test	Dosage per animal (mg)	% Animals ovulating	Mean no. of eggs	Inhibition of ovulation[a]
Equanil	30	0.3	60	7.0	+
		3.0	20	0.8	++
		5.0	0	0	+++
Sparine	20	0.1	60	11.8	+
		0.5	0	0	+++
Chlorpromazine	30	0.01	60	6.4	+
		0.125	20	2.2	++
		0.25	0	0	+++
Atarax	20	0.1	80	14.6	
		1.0	20	4.0	++
Trilafon	20	0.01	100	22.8	
		0.1	0	0	+++
Paxitol	20	0.1	80	17.6	
		1.0	0	0	+++
Compazine	20	0.1	60	11.0	+
		1.0	0	0	+++
Stelazine	20	0.02	80	21.8	
		0.20	20	2.4	++
Atropine	10	0.04	60	5.4	+
		0.4	0	0	+++
Metropine	10	0.25	80	14.0	
		0.5	40	3.6	+
Demerol	10	0.02	100	25.4	
		0.2	60	13.8	
Phenobarbital	10	0.10	60	17.6	
		1.0	40	6.0	+
Dibenamine	10	0.05	80	8.2	+
		0.5	20	1.4	++
Benadryl	10	0.10	60	16.8	
		0.5	60	6.8	+
Estrone	10	0.10	100	20.8	
		1.0	80	7.8	+
17α-Ethynylestradiol-3- methyl ether	10	0.01	80	15.4	
		0.05	80	7.8	+
Cortisone	10	0.3	80	12.2	
		3.0	40	4.8	+
Progesterone	10	0.25	60	5.8	+
		0.5	0	0	+++

TABLE 11 (*Continued*)

Compound	No. animals in test	Dosage per animal (mg)	% Animals ovulating	Mean no. of eggs	Inhibition of ovulation[a]
17α-Ethyl-19-nortesto-	10	0.10	100	22.6	
sterone		0.50	80	17.2	
17α-Ethynyl estra-$\Delta^{5(10)}$-	10	0.15	50	11.6	
enolone		1.50	10	1.6	++
17α-Methylallyl-19-nor-	10	0.10	100	19.2	
testosterone		1.50	80	4.0	+
6α-Chloro-17-acetoxy-	10	0.50	100	17.8	
progesterone		2.0	40	5.2	+

[a] + indicates significant reduction in number of eggs; ++, significant reduction in both ovulation rate and number of eggs; and +++, complete suppression of ovulation.

(*309*). The optimal ovulating regime was found to be the intraperitoneal injection of 2 IU of pregnant mare's serum (PMS) followed 42 hours later by intraperitoneal human chorionic gonadotropin (HCG) and autopsy for counting of ova 20 hours later. An average of 28 eggs in the mouse are produced. The administration of potential inhibitors could be made at any time, but ordinarily preceding HCG. In Table 11 are the data obtained on a variety of compounds tested. When ten animals are tested a statistically significant effect is had when the percentage ovulating is 40 or less, or the number of eggs ovulated is 14 or less. It may be seen that at rather elevated doses every steroid tested significantly reduced the mean number of ova ovulated, but that a number of CNS depressants were active at lower doses. Actually the most active compound proved to be reserpine; at 0.01 mg per mouse it reduces the ovulation percentages to 40 and the mean egg number to 4. The implication of this procedure is that the direct effect of exogenous gonadotropin on ovarian follicles is inhibited. A possible "activation" of the animals' endogenous gonadotropin-secreting mechanism necessary for the complete action of exogenous gonadotropin is not obviated. The various active agents then inhibit this endogenous mechanism (*310*) which presumably is centrally located. Superovulation induced by PMS alone in immature rats may be

inhibited by hypophysectomy or by Dibenamine, atropine, SKF-
501, and Nembutal (311). Zarrow and Quinn conclude that PMS
acting on the ovary produces an agent that stimulates endogenous
LH via a central mechanism. Aron and Asch (312) claim that this
central mechanism is activated by coitus in the rat and that the
released neurohumor is cholinergic. The involvement of a cholinergic mechanism is also suggested by Quinn and Zarrow (313).
Since serotonin administration to PMS-treated immature rats either
during or after PMS administration prevented ovarian luteinization
a serotonin-labile LHRF releasing mechanism is activated by the
PMS regimen (314). When exogenous LH is substituted for HCG
in the induction of superovulation in immature rats there is no
increase in the ovarian RNA:DNA ratio seen with HCG, nor does
progesterone inhibit the LH-induced superovulation although it is
partially inhibitory to the HCG superovulation (315). Suggestive
of an inhibitory hypothalamic mechanism is the finding that a rat
hypothalamus extract injected at 49 hours after PMS administration
to rats inhibits the superovulation (316).

Edgren and Carter (317) have found that HCG-induced ovulation in the rabbit cannot be blocked by the administration of
steroids that inhibit copulation-induced ovulation. Furthermore,
compounds clearly inhibitory in mice, e.g., progesterone and norethynodrel, were not inhibitory in HCG-injected rabbits. Again we
appear to be faced with the possibility of species differences in
mechanisms involved, although in the adult rabbit and immature
mouse these responsivities may devolve on different bases, e.g.,
follicle rupture in the rabbit; follicle growth in the mouse.

Barbiturate may inhibit PMS-induced ovulation in the 31-day-
old rat when administered at 2:00 to 4:00 P.M., 48 hours after PMS
injection (318). In preliminary studies we have found that reserpine
and other tranquilizers are also effective at rather limited times
in PMS-HCG-ovulated rats (319). This ovulation-inhibiting action
has previously been observed in the adult rat [166, 170 (Ch. 3)]
where it is adjudged a blockade of gonadotropin release. A potent
oral reserpate (SU 7064) has been found to be a most active sup-
pressor of estrus in the rat with few side effects (320). Ovulation
inhibition in the monkey by reserpine has also been reported (209).

In reporting on further studies of the effects of ataractic drugs on superovulation in mice, Purshottam (*310*) noted that their anti-ovulatory activity paralleled their sedative action and concluded that superovulation in immature mice involved a hypothalamic activation. Reserpine, but no other tranquilizer, will, however, inhibit PMS-HCG ovulation in hypophysectomized rats (*319*). Direct action of this agent on the ovarian follicle thus seems certain. The steroids remain to be studied in detail in such hypophysectomized preparations, but cortisol has been especially effective and estrogens partially effective (*321*).

Miscellaneous Antigonadotropic Agents

A method of ovulation inhibition that has received some attention involves the use of processes or agents that might inactivate circulating gonadotropin. The most outstanding example is a gonadotropin inhibitor present in extracts of *Lithospermum ruderale*. Inactivation of gonadotropin *in vitro* by such extracts was originally demonstrated (*322*) and a fairly stable powder containing the activity also acts *in vivo* (*323*). Fractionation of extracts has led to the isolation of crystalline and noncrystalline constituents (*324*), but there is also a tendency for the desired activity to disappear. The latest word by one of the most active workers with this material is: "Extensive attempts have been made to determine the mode of action and isolate the active constituent, but the problems involved seem complex and the present state of the matter is unsatisfactory" (*325*). A substance called lithospermum is present in *Lathyrus odoratus* extracts; it appears to interfere with estrogen and progestin production by the ovaries rather than with ovulation but its possible action in this regard is not obviated [*42* (Ch. 2), *326*]. Another plant yielding an antigonadotropic extract is *Lycopus virginicus*, the extract of which appears to be most potent as an antithyrotropin (*327*).

Other gonadotropin-inhibiting preparations have been described. They include enzyme-like inactivators such as lysozyme which is active *in vivo* against hypophyseal and human chorionic gonadotropin (*328*). Since lysozyme does not inhibit gonadotropin-induced ovulation in rabbits and produces a transient genitourinary blockage to sperm discharge in frogs, its importance as a true antigonadotropin has been questioned (329).

A synthetic agent that has antifertility effects is a dithiocarbamoylhydrazine (ICI-33,828) which inhibits pituitary gonadotropic function in rats and mice (330, 331). Apparently it may have a dual effect since (a) its sterilizing action is accompanied by a decrease of pituitary FSH and (b) it may modify the animals' response to exogenous gonadotropin (331). The possibility of an effect on target organs to pituitary hormones is illustrated by its action as an inhibitor of growth hormone action on the tibia and on general growth in hypophysectomized rats (332), but direct *in vivo* neutralization is not excluded since it inhibits growth or may even cause weight loss in intact animals (331). Indeed suppression of TSH (333) and lactogenic hormones (334) by this agent is indicated.

Rather mysterious effects on ovulation have been reported for propylthiouracil (PTU) which in rats decreases the number of ova produced to zero in females having it in the feed to 0.05% (334). In superovulated mice, on the other hand, PTU feeding causes an increase in the number of ova and *l*-thyroxine a decrease (335). Even more mysterious is the effect of chloroguanidine at a concentration of 0.005 to 0.025% in the diet of female mice. It prevents fertility and the only visible sign of its action is an increase in the number of corpora lutea. It has no antifertility effect in male mice, and two related compounds, phenformin and abityl guanidine, which act like it on malarial parasites, have no antifertility effects in either male or female mice (336).

Endogenously produced antigonadotropins may originate in the pituitary itself. This is suggested by the finding that crude preparations of pituitary FSH and LH inhibit the gonadotropic potency of PMS and HCG in test animals whereas, with purification, particularly of FSH, this antagonistic action disappeared. Furthermore, the greater efficacy of subcutaneous FSH over intraperitoneal FSH diminished with continued purification of FSH, indicating the loss of an accompanying inhibitor (337).

Another endogenous mammalian antigonadotropin is suggested by the presence in fetal serum, but not in normal serum, of an inhibitor of HCG activity (*338*). An antigonadotropic activity of pineal extracts has been described (*339*) and it has been claimed that this inhibitory "pineal hormone" may be extracted from the urine of children (*340*). It is found in the supernatant of a TCA (trichloro acetic acid) precipitate of cattle pineal glands and inhibits the action of exogenous and endogenous gonadotropin (*341*). A similar material has been indicated as occurring in the serum of mentally and physically retarded children (*342*). The presumed pineal factor has been called "anestrin" since it is antigonadotropic in female and not in male rats (*343*). Since 5-methoxytryptophal, a probable metabolite of melatonin, is antigonadotropic in immature rats and melatonin is present in pineal glands, pineal methoxy indoles have been suggested as the active pineal material (*344*). An antigonadotropic agent present in children's urine and which acts against HCG but not against estrogen has been described by Soffer *et al.* (*345*). More recent study has revealed the presence of this agent in adults' urine at all ages. It is a heat-stable substance insoluble in either 95% ethanol or ether (*346*). It fails to inhibit FSH or menopausal gonadotropin effects in immature mice, but inhibits pituitary LH action in the ventral prostate test in hypophysectomized rats (*347, 348*). A nonlipid, nonprotein, water-soluble, dialyzable, thermolabile, anti-FSH substance has been prepared from bovine serum (*349*).

No account of attempts at ovulation control can be complete without some mention of attempts to employ gonadotropins as antibodies. That antibodies to gonadotropic preparations may be obtained was long ago established (cf. *350, 351*). These are interspecific immunities which generally are directed against species-specific protein rather than against the protein or polypeptide hormone as such [*179* (Ch. 3), *352*]. The search, therefore, is for gonadotropin-specific antibodies (*353*), and there has been some suggestion of progress toward the attainment of this objective. Thus rabbit antiserum to sheep pituitary LH inhibited not only the action in rats of administered sheep LH (*359*) but of endogenous LH in young rats and the action of PMS and human LH in test hypophysectomized male rats. LH derived from rat, pig, and whole pituitaries was acted against by this rabbit antiserum, but neither HCG nor chicken "LH" activity was affected (*354*). Similarly, guinea pig pituitary gonadotropin-induced antiserum from rabbits acted as an antigonadotropin in mice as well as guinea pigs (356). This rabbit antiserum appeared to effect specific hypophyseal lesions in the guinea pig (357). When HCG is used as an antigen, immunity to FSH, ICSH, and HCG may be had (354). Rabbit antiserum to ovine LH will inhibit ovulation in cycling rats if injected 12 hours before an expected ovulation, but no inhibition of vaginal estrus occurs (358). On the other hand, antiserum to PMS produced in hamsters will not inhibit ovum release but will prevent the superovulating action of PMS (355). Much remains to be done in this area relative not only to specific immunity to specific gonadotropins, but also to duration of immunity, chemical nature of the antibodies, factors influencing their operation, and so on (see 353, 361).

An attempt to use steroids as haptenes in synthetic antigens has thus far not led to the development of significant reactions against endogenous steroid hormone (362), but preinjection will prevent exogenous hormone (estrogenic, androgenic, corticoid) effects in standard assays (363).

REFERENCES

206. Benoit, J., and Assenmacher, I. 1955. *J. Physiol.* (*Paris*) **47,** 427.
207. Everett, J. W. 1944. *Endocrinology* **35,** 507.
208. Meier, R. L. 1959. "Modern Science and the Human Fertility Problem." Wiley, New York.
209. DeFoe, V. J., and Reynolds, S. R. M. 1956. *Science* **124,** 726.
210. Pasteels, J. L. 1961. *Ann. Endocrinol.* **22,** 257.
211. Ratner, A., and Meites, J. 1964. *Federation Proc.* **23,** 110.
212. Kanematsu, S., Hilliard, J., and Sawyer, C. H. 1963. *Acta Endocrinol.* **44,** 467.
213. Barraclough, C. A. 1956. *Anat. Record* **124,** 255.
214. Velardo, J. T. 1958. *Fertility Sterility* **9,** 60.
215. Jarrett, R. J. 1963. *Brit. J. Pharmacol.* **20,** 497.
216. Talwalker, P. K., Meites, J., Nicoll, C. S., and Hopkins, T. F. 1960. *Am. J. Physiol.* **199,** 1073.
217. Kahn, M. Y. 1962. *Anat. Record* **142,** 248.
218. Gitsch, E., and Everett, J. W. 1958. *Endocrinology* **62,** 400.
219. Mayer, G., Thevenot-Duluc, A. J., and Meunier, J. M. 1961. *Compt. Rend. Soc. Biol.* **155,** 1285.
220. Harris, G. W. 1961. *In* "Control of Ovulation" (C. A. Villee, ed.), p. 56. Pergamon Press, New York.

221. Sawyer, C. H., and Kawakami, M. 1961. *In* "Control of Ovulation" (C. A. Villee, ed.), p. 79. Pergamon Press, New York.
222. Szontagh, F. E., and Uhlark, S. 1964. *J. Endocrinol.* **29**, 203.
223. McCann, S. M., and Taleisnik, S. 1961. *Endocrinology* **68**, 1071.
224. McCann, S. M., and Ramirez, V. D. 1962. *Proc. 1st Intern. Congr. Hormonal Steroids, Milan*, p. 25.
225. Donnet, V., Chevalier, J. M., Duflot, J. C., and Jacquin, M. 1962. *Compt. Rend. Soc. Biol.* **156**, 1123.
226. Fevold, H. L., Hisaw, F. L., and Greep, R. O. 1936. *Am. J. Physiol.* **117**, 68.
227. Suzuki, M., Hirano, M., Kobayashi, M., and Nakano, M. 1961. *J. Japan Obstet. Gynecol. Soc.* **8**, 47.
228. Hilliard, J., and Sawyer, C. H. 1962. *Proc. 1st Intern. Congr. Hormonal Steroids, Milan*, p. 26.
229. Suzuki, M., and Bialy, G. 1964. *Endocrinology* **74**, 780.
230. Kincl, F. A. 1963 *Endokrinologie* **44**, 67.
231. Everett, J. W., Radford, H. M., and Holsinger, J. 1962. *Proc. 1st Intern. Congr. Hormonal Steroids, Milan* p. 24.
232. Everett, J. W. 1964. *In* "Major Problems in Neuroendocrinology" (E. Bajusz and G. Jasmir, eds.), p. 346. S. Karger, Basel.
233. Critchlow, V. 1958. *Am. J. Physiol.* **195**, 171.
234. Pincus, G., Chang, M. C., Zarrow, M. X., Hafez, E. S. E., and Merrill, A. P. 1956. *Endocrinology* **59**, 695.
235. Kincl, F. A., and Dorfman, R. I. 1963. *Acta Endocrinol. Suppl.* **73**, 3.
236. Kincl, F. A., and Dorfman, R. I. 1963. *Acta Endocrinol. Suppl.* **73**, 17.
237. Lutwak-Mann, C. 1955. *J. Endocrinol.* **13**, 26.
238. Pincus, G., Miyake, T., Merrill, A. P., and Longo, P. 1957. *Endocrinology* **61**, 528.
239. Ogawa, Y., and Pincus, G. 1961. *Endocrinology* **68**, 680.
240. Miyake, T. 1962. *In* "Methods in Hormone Research" (R. I. Dorfman, ed.), Vol. II, p. 129. Academic Press, New York.
241. Van der Werff ten Bosh, J. J. 1961. *Medicamunde* **7**, 109.
242. Falconi, G., Gardi, R., Bruni, G., and Ercoli, A. 1961. *Endocrinology* **69**, 638.
243. Verna, F., and Castiglione, C. 1962. *Minerva Ginecol.* **14/17**, 861.
244. Shipley, E. 1962. *In* "Methods in Hormone Research" (R. I. Dorfman, ed.), Vol. II, p. 179. Academic Press, New York.
245. Burrows, H. 1949. "Biological Actions of Sex Hormones," 2nd ed. Cambridge Univ. Press, London and New York.
246. Byrnes, W. W., and Meyer, R. K. 1951. *Endocrinology* **49**, 449.
247. Greep, R. O., and Chester Jones, I. 1950. *Recent Progr. Hormone Res.* **5**, 197.
248. Byrnes, W. W., Meyer, R. K., and Finerty, J. D. 1951. *Am. J. Physiol.* **164**, 26.
249. Perrine, J. W. 1961. *Acta Endocrinol.* **37**, 376.
250. Falconi, G., and Bruni, G. 1962. *J. Endocrinol.* **25**, 169.

251. Dorfman, R. I., Caspi, E., and Grover, P. K. 1962. *Proc. Soc. Exptl. Biol. Med.* **110**, 750.
252. Miyake, T. 1961. *Endocrinology* **69**, 534.
253. Lipschutz, A., Iglesias, R., and Salinas, S. 1962. *Nature* **196**, 946.
254. Saunders, F. J. 1958. *Endocrinology* **63**, 561.
255. Goisis, M., and Mosca, L. 1962. *Quart. J. Exptl. Physiol.* **47**, 299.
256. Gans, E., and Van Rees, G. P. 1962. *Acta Endocrinol.* **39**, 245.
257. Mangili, G., Martini, L., and Pecile, A. 1961. *Folia Endocrinol.* **14**, 377.
258. Bancale, E., Giuliani, G., and Mangili, G. 1960. *Atti Accad. Med. Lombarda* **15**, 55.
259. Flerko, B. 1962. *Proc. 1st Intern. Congr. Hormonal Steroids, Milan* p. 23.
260. Davidson, J. M., and Sawyer, C. H. 1961. *Acta Endocrinol.* **37**, 385.
261. Kanematsu, S., and Sawyer, C. H. 1962. *Endocrinology* **72**, 243.
262. Lisk, R. D. 1962. *Acta Endocrinol.* **41**, 195.
263. Desclin, L., Flament-Durand, J., and Gepts, W. 1962. *Endocrinology* **70**, 429.
264. Bogdanove, E. M. 1963. *Endocrinology* **73**, 696.
265. Nikitovitch-Winer, M. B. 1962. *Endocrinology* **70**, 350.
266. Nedde, N. P., and Nikitovitch-Winer, M. B. 1964. *Anat. Record* **148**, 317.
267. Courrier, R., Guillemin, R., Justisz, M., Sakiz, E., and Aschheim, P. 1961. *Compt. Rend. Acad Sci.* **253**, 922.
268. Schiavi, R., Justisz, M., Sakiz, E., and Guillemin, R. 1963. *Proc. Soc. Exptl. Biol. Med.* **114**, 426.
269. Igarashi, M., Nallar, R., Ramirez, V. D., and McCann, S. M. 1964. *Federation Proc.* **23**, 151.
270. Clark, G. 1942. *Am. J. Physiol.* **137**, 746.
271. Bogdanove, E. M., and Halmi, N. S. 1953. *Endocrinology* **53**, 274.
272. Szentagothai, J., Flerko, B., Mess, S., and Halasz, B. 1962. Akademia Kiado. Budapest.
273. Kennedy, G. C., and Mitra, J. 1963. *J. Physiol. (London)* **166**, 395.
274. Averill, R. W. L., and Purves, H. D. 1963. *J. Endocrinol.* **26**, 463.
275. Domingo, R. V., and McCann, S. M. 1963. *Endocrinology* **73**, 193.
276. McCann, S. M., and Ramirez, V. D. 1964. *Rec. Progr. Hormone Res.* **20**, 131.
277. Everett, J. W. 1961. *In* "Control of Ovulation" (C. A. Villee, ed.), p. 101. Pergamon Press, New York.
278. Bar-Sela, M. E. 1964. *Anat. Record* **148**, 359.
279. Nalbandov, A. V. 1961. *In* "Control of Ovulation" (C. A. Villee, ed.), p. 122. Pergamon Press, New York.
280. Smedik, P. G., and Sawyer, C. H. 1962. *Acta Endocrinol.* **41**, 561.
281. Martini, L., Fochi, M., Gavazzi, G., and Pecile, A. 1962. *Arch. Intern. Pharmacodyn.* **140**, 156.
282. Barraclough, C. A., and Gorski, R. A. 1962. *J. Endocrinol.* **25**, 175.
283. Palka, Y. S., and Sawyer, C. H. 1964. *Am. Zool.* **4**, 289.

284. Taleisnik, S., Caligaris, L., and De Olmos, J. 1962. *Am. J. Physiol.* **203**, 1109.

285. Conrey, K., and de Groot, J. 1964. *Federation Proc.* **23**, 109.

286. Hayward, J. N., Hilliard, J., and Sawyer, C. H. 1964. *Endocrinology* **74**, 108.

287. Parlow, A. F. 1964. *Rec. Progr. Hormone Res.* **20**, 171.

288. Overbeek, G. A., and de Visser, J. 1964. *Acta Endocrinol. Suppl.* **90**, 179.

289. Kanematsu, S., and Sawyer, C. H. 1963. *Endocrinology* **73**, 687.

290. Kato, J. 1963. *Endocrinol. Japon.* **10**, 145.

291. Kobayashi, T., Kobayashi, T., Kato, J., and Minaguchi, H. 1964. *Endocrinol. Japon.* **11**, 9.

292. Sala, G. 1962. *Proc. 1st Intern. Congr. Hormonal Steroids, Milan* p. 11.

293. Steelman, S. L., Oslapas, R., Morgan, E. R., and Busch, R. D. 1962. *Federation Proc.* **21**, 213.

294. Lerner, L. J., Yiacas, E., Bianchi, A., Turkheimer, A. R., De Phillipo, M., and Borman, A. 1962. *Proc. 1st Intern. Congr. Hormonal Steroids, Milan* p. 188.

295. Lerner, L. J., Yiacas, E., Bianchi, A., Turkheimer, A. R., De Phillipo, M., and Borman, A. 1964. *Fertility Sterility* **15**, 63.

296. Hartley, F. 1962. *J. Endocrinol.* **24**, xvi.

297. David, A., Edwards, K., Fellowes, K. P., and Plummer, J. M. 1963. *J. Reprod. Fertility* **5**, 331.

298. Edgren, R. A., Smith, H., Peterson, D. L., and Carter, D. L. 1963. *Steroids* **2**, 319.

299. Duncan, G. W., Lyster, S. C., and Campbell, J. A. 1964. *Proc. Soc. Exptl. Biol. Med.* **116**, 800.

300. Schoeler, H. F. L. 1963. *J. Reprod. Fertility* **5**, 455.

301. Bradbury, J. T. 1961. *Endocrinology* **68**, 115.

302. Aron, C., Asch, G., and Asch, L. 1962. *Arch. Anat. Microscop. Morphol. Exptl.* **51**, 27.

303. Holmes, R. L., and Mandl, A. M. 1962. *J. Endocrinol.* **24**, 497.

304. Saunders, F. J., and Drill, V. A. 1958. *Ann. N. Y. Acad. Sci.* **71**, 516.

305. Eckstein, P., and Mandl, A. M. 1962. *Endocrinology* **71**, 964.

306. Wright, P. A. 1960. *Biol. Bull.* **119**, 351.

307. Kullander, S. 1961. *Acta Endocrinol.* **38**, 598.

308. Kar, A. B., Mundle, M., and Roy, S. 1960. *J. Sci. Ind. Res.* **19C**, 264.

309. Purshottam, N., Mason, M. M., and Pincus, G. 1961. *Fertility Sterility* **12**, 346.

310. Purshottam, N. 1962. *Am. J. Obstet. Gynecol.* **83**, 1405.

311. Zarrow, M. X., and Quinn, D. L. 1963. *J. Endocrinol.* **26**, 181.

312. Aron, C., and Asch, G. 1962. *Compt. Rend. Acad. Sci.* **255**, 3056.

313. Quinn, D. L., and Zarrow, M. X. 1964. *Endocrinology* **74**, 309.

314. O'Steen, W. K. 1964. *Endocrinology* **74**, 885.

315. Callantine, M. R., Lee, S. L., Humphrey, R., and Windsor, B. 1964. *Federation Proc.* **23**, 463.

316. Hopkins, T. F., and Pincus, G. 1964. *Federation Proc.* 23, 411.
317. Edgren, R. A., and Carter, D. L. 1962. *J. Endocrinol.* 24, 525.
318. Strauss, W. F., and Meyer, R. K. 1962. *Science* 137, 860.
319. Hopkins, T. F., and Pincus, G. 1963. *Federation Proc.* 22, 506.
320. Gaunt, R., Renzi, A. A., and Chart, J. J. 1962. *Endocrinology* 71, 527.
321. France, E., and Pincus, G. 1964. *Endocrinology* 75, 359.
322. Noble, R. L., Plunkett, E. R., and Graham, R. C. B. 1954. *J. Endocrinol.* 10, 212.
323. Breneman, W. R., and Carmack, M. 1958. *Anat. Record* 131, 538.
324. Gorman, M., Bien, S., and Ginsburg, D. 1956. *Bull. Res. Council Israel* 5, 253.
325. Noble, R. L. 1959. *Proc. 6th Intern. Conf. Planned Parenthood, New Delhi, India,* p. 243.
326. Walker, J., and Wirtschafter, Z. 1956. *J. Nutr.* 58, 161.
327. Kemper, F., and Loeser, A. 1961. *Acta Endocrinol.* 38, 200.
328. Albano, S. B., and Carollo, F. 1960. *Boll. Soc. Ital. Biol. Sper.* 36, 1142.
329. Sermann, R. 1961. *Minerva Ginecol.* 13, 1266.
330. Brown, P. S. 1963. *J. Endocrinol.* 26, 425.
331. Benson, G. K. 1964. *J. Endocrinol.* 58, ix.
332. Thompson, H. E. C. G. 1963. *J. Endocrinol.* 26, 447.
333. Tulloch, M. I., Crooks, J., and Brown, P. S. 1963. *Nature* 199, 288.
334. Wilson, E. D., Runner, M. N., and Zarrow, M. X. 1963. *J. Reprod. Fertility* 5, 233.
335. Wilson, E. D., and Chai, C. K. 1962. *J. Endocrinol.* 24, 431.
336. Cutting, W. 1962. *Antibiot. Chemotherapy* 12, 671.
337. Woods, M. C., and Simpson, M. E. 1961. *Endocrinology* 68, 647.
338. Casaglia, G., and Foggioli, A. 1961. *Boll. Soc. Ital. Biol. Sper.* 37, 60.
339. Bianchini, P., and Osima, B. 1960. *Atti Accad. Med. Lombarda* 15, 101.
340. Milcu, I., Damion, E., and Ionesen, M. 1960. *Studii Cercetari Endocrinol.* 11, 651.
341. Reiss, M., Davis, R. H., Sideman, M. B., Mauer, I., and Plichta, E. S. 1963. *J. Endocrinol.* 27, 107.
342. Reiss, M., Pearse, J. J., Davis, R. H., Hillman, J. C., and Sideman, M. B. 1964. *J. Endocrinol.* 29, 83.
343. Bianchini, P., and Osima, B. 1963. *Boll. Soc. Ital. Biol. Sper.* 38, 1547.
344. McIsaac, W. M., Taborsky, R. G., and Farrell, G. 1964. *Science* 145, 63.
345. Soffer, L. J., Futterweit, W., and Salvaneschi, J. 1961. *J. Clin. Endocrinol. Metab.* 21, 1267.
346. Soffer, L. J., Salvaneschi, J., and Futterweit, W. 1962. *J. Clin. Endocrinol. Metab.* 22, 532.
347. Soffer, L. J., and Fogel, M. 1963. *J. Clin. Endocrinol.* 23, 870.
348. Futterweit, W., Margolis, S., Soffer, L. J., and Dorfman, R. I. 1963. *Endocrinology* 72, 903.
349. Fachin, G., Toffoli, C., Gaudiano, A., Marabelli, M., and Polizzi, M. 1963. *Nature* 199, 195.

350. Zondek, B., and Sulman, F. 1942. "The Antigonadotrophic Factor, with Consideration of the Antihormone Problem." Williams & Wilkins, Baltimore, Maryland.

351. Leathem, J. H. 1949. *Recent Progr. Hormone Res.* **4**, 115.

352. Geschwind, I. I. 1959. *In* "Comparative Endocrinology" (A. Gorbman, ed.), p. 421. Wiley, New York.

353. Segal, S. J. 1962. *In* "Research in Family Planning" (Kiser, ed.), p. 337. Princeton Univ. Press, Princeton, New Jersey.

354. Moudgal, N. R., and Li, C. H. 1961. *Arch. Biochem.* **95**, 93.

355. Greenwald, G. S. 1963. *Anat. Record* **145**, 235.

356. Loth, G., Montale, P., and Azzena, D. 1960. *Boll. Soc. Ital. Biol. Sper.* **36**, 1192.

357. Cacioppo, A., Azzena, D., and Montale, P. 1960. *Arch. Maragliano Patol. Clin.* **16**, 783.

358. Kelly, W. A., Robertson, H. A., and Stanisfield, D. A. 1963. *J. Endocrinol.* **27**, 127.

359. Bourdel, G. 1961. *Gen. Comp. Endocrinol.* **1**, 375.

360. Isersky, C., Lunenfeld, B., and Shelesnyak, M. C. 1962. *Life Sci.* **7**, 337.

361. Segal, S. J., Laurence, K. A., Perlbachs, M., and Hakim, S. 1962. *Gen. Comp. Endocrinol. Suppl.* **1**, 12.

362. Lieberman, S., Erlanger, B. F., Beiser, S. M., and Agate, F. J., Jr. 1959. *Recent Progr. Hormone Res.* **15**, 165.

363. Neri, R. O., Tolksdorf, S. M., Beiser, S. M., Erlanger, B. F., Agate, F. J., Jr., and Lieberman, S. 1964. *Endocrinology* **74**, 593.

CHAPTER 5

Fertilization

Recent detailed accounts of the observable events taking place at fertilization, the reactions occurring in sperm and ova, and of the hypotheses advanced to account for these reactions, are those of Austin [9 (Ch. 1)], Bishop [51 (Ch. 2)], Blandau [89 (Ch. 2)], and Tyler [179 (Ch. 3)]. Ideally, one should be able to define in physical terms the requirements put upon sperm and ova so that they may successfully effect fertilization and the consequent ovum cleavage. These requirements are only partially known; many allegedly essential conditions have proven controversial, and the limitations to quantitative study in mammals of what appears to be a complex series of sequential steps have often led to the appearance of problems before the attainment of solutions.

We have already indicated that before ovum penetration by sperm is achieved a degree of maturation of both gametes appears to be essential. Thus, in practically all mammals the freshly ovulated ova have already had a first maturation division with the formation of the first polar body. In the rabbit, the processes leading to first polar body extrusion are initiated by mating or following intravenous administration of gonadotropin and are concluded by the eighth hour postcoitum (364). Because the intrafollicular microinjection of chorionic gonadotropin in minute amount was followed in several instances by polar body formation, a direct action of gonadotropin on either follicular fluid or the ovum has been postulated (365), despite the demonstration that isolating the ovum from the follicle (e.g., in culture *in vitro*) is enough to cause such maturation (*364*). Sperm capacitation for fertilization has been described previously. Since evidence of capacitation is thus far had for certain mammalian species (rabbit, rat, hamster, and sheep) (*366*) but not for others (mouse, guinea pig, man), Blandau [89 (Ch. 2)] has stated: "There has been much speculation on the importance of capacitation in fertilization, but there is little significant evidence to support the various theories proposed." Nonetheless, this phenomenon appears to have been essential to the most convincing instance of mammalian ovum fertilization *in vitro*. By taking capacitated sperm from the rabbit uterus at 12 hours postcoitum and incubating them with rabbit ova for 3 to 4 hours, Chang (*367*) was able to culture the ova to cleavage and to secure viable young from them following transplantation to foster mothers. Previous attempts by a number of other workers over a number of years to demonstrate unequivocally fertilization *in vitro* (cf. *368*) led either to failure or equivocal results due to the possibility of occurrence of parthenogenetic activation or of cleavage-simulating cytoplasm fragmentation rather than true fertilization. In any event, it is certain that procedures inhibiting rabbit sperm capacitation such as the pseudopregnant state or progesterone administration [82 (Ch. 2)] or certain constituents of plasma (*369*) prevent fertilization [cf. 78 (Ch. 2)].

The concept originally advanced by Austin [9 (Ch.1)] that capacitation is the loss of the acrosome cap would suggest that measures preventing acrosome cap loss might be fertilization-inhibiting. However, rabbit sperm do not lose the cap until entry into the zona pellucida and perivitelline space has been accomplished (*370*). Furthermore, a study of mouse semen in aged animals discloses a decreasing percentage of the relatively infertile sperm with normal caps (*371*), and the progressive loss of acrosome caps observed in a proportion of rabbit sperm after ejaculation has been termed not capacitation but a "manifestation of a senile state" in a proportion of the sperm population (*372*). Finally, Chang (*369*) has shown a reversibility of capacitation in the rabbit by immersing capacitated sperm in dilute seminal plasma. Austin (*373*) has therefore suggested that capacitation is a two-stage phenomenon: (a) the removal of a stabilizing substance making possible (b) the physiological changes associated with acrosome modification; Chang's reversal of capacitation could then be attributed to the acquisition of the stabilizer.

The often demonstrated inhibition of sperm-fertility capacity simply as the result of exposure to the medium in which eggs have been placed has led, often by devious steps, to the concept of fertilization as analogous to an immunity reaction. The active substance produced by eggs is fertilizin. As produced by sea urchin eggs, it is a gel-forming glycoprotein with a molecular weight of approximately 300,000. According to the theory of Lillie (374), of which Tyler (375) is the chief present-day proponent, fertilizin located in the egg plasma membrane acts as a receptor for antifertilizin, a protein located on the surface of spermatozoa. It is the union of fertilizin and antifertilizin which is the functional event of fertilization and which is responsible for characteristic changes in cortical viscosity, the inhibition of polyspermy, various metabolic processes culminating in second polar body formation, and so on. It is fertilizin present in excess in media containing eggs that causes sperm often to agglutinate and always to lose fertilizing capacity. Reversal of agglutination (which often occurs spontaneously) does not lead to recovery of fertilizing capacity, but washing a sperm suspension so as to remove fertilizin from its binding by antifertilizin may restore fertilizing capacity. Although most of the work on this mechanism of fertilization has been conducted in nonmammalian animals, the phenomenon of agglutination by mammalian egg products has been described (376), and the washing of rabbit eggs, presumably thereby removing excess fertilizin, has increased the percentage of successful fertilizations *in vitro* (377). Just as excess fertilizin inhibits sperm-fertilizing capacity, so excess antifertilizin prevents eggs from being fertilized. Thus far neither fertilizin nor antifertilizin have been employed experimentally in mammals as agents for fertility control. Their protein nature would seem to preclude their parenteral use, and their antigenic activity seems to make imperative the search for species-specific fertilizins and antifertilizins. However, an inquiry into agents and processes affecting their concentrations in the gametes and their union may very well reveal readily useful antifertility agents.

Unfortunately the problem is not simplified by the findings of species differences among mammals in the presumed basic fertilization reactions. Thus Thibault and Dauzier (378) find the removal of fertilizin from rabbit eggs (by washing for 2 hours in Locke's solution) removes the bar to capacitated sperm penetration *in vitro*. They find that *in vivo* an antifertilizin produced presumably by the Fallopian tubes neutralizes ovum fertilizin. Neither ewe nor sow ova could be fertilized *in vitro* using procedures designed to remove or neutralize ovum-generated fertilizin. We have indicated that a parthenogenetic activation might result simply by explantation of ova and this might prevent normal fertilization (and explain the lack of success with ewe and sow ova). However, Chalmel (379) has found that rabbit ova parthenogenetically activated by exposure to cold may indeed be penetrated by sperm either *in vivo* or *in vitro*. Since polyspermy is rare in such ova we have here the bar to supernumerary sperm which is one of the features of normal fertilization. Abortive segmentation of these ova indicates, however, a block to normal development.

Two other processes involving sperm in the female reproductive tract have led to experiments concerned with eventual fertilizing capacity. The first of these is sperm agglutination due to a large number of factors other than fertilizin, e.g., specific ions, pH variations, degrees of salinity (cf. 380). The second is hyaluronic acid depolymerization by the sperm-borne enzyme hyaluronidase. The rather nonspecific sperm agglutination may be inhibited by antagglutins present in prostatic and follicular fluids and in secretions of the Fallopian tubes and of the cervix (381, 382) and Lindahl believes that normal fertilization is made possible by their presence in semen and in female reproductive tract fluids. He has advanced the notion that the antibodies to these "natural" antagglutins may act as antifertility agents (383). Full demonstration of this possibility remains to be made.

The hyaluronidase activity of sperm has indeed been examined in some detail experimentally as a basis for altering fertility. In our original studies of the follicle cell-dispersing activity of rabbit sperm *in vitro*, we pointed out that some 20,000 sperm per cubic centimeter were needed to effect a significant breakdown of the intracellular cement (384). This led to the concept that a "sperm swarm" was needed in the oviducts to produce an amount of hyaluronidase sufficient to remove the often dense mass of follicle cells surrounding freshly ovulated ova before the penetrating spermatozoon could reach the egg. It is now generally recognized that the number of sperm at the site of fertilization in mammals is quite low, and very much less than the thousands found necessary for follicle cell dispersion. This is evident from the data collected in Table 12 [51 (Ch. 2)]. Furthermore, careful examination of

TABLE 12

Number of Spermatozoa Found at the Site of
Fertilization in Several Mammals[a]

Species	Mean no. of sperm per tube	Postcoital time (hr)	Reference
Rat	43	?	385
	12	12	386
	30	24	
	45	12	387, 388
Mouse	17	10–15	387
Rabbit	500	?	389
	38	4	390
	250	10	
Ferret	200	6	84 (Ch. 2)
Sheep	500	24	
	184[b]	24–48	387
	673[c]	24–48	

[a] From Bishop [51 (Ch. 2)].
[b] Ovarian third of oviduct.
[c] Entire ampulla.

freshly fertilized mammalian eggs has shown that sperm penetration into the egg may occur before any significant dispersal of the major follicle cell mass [7 (Ch. 1), 89 (Ch. 2), 391, 393]. Therefore, it would seem that liberation of hyaluronidase into the intratubal "culture" of follicle cells cum ova is not a necessity for fertilization, nor indeed a very likely usual event. The penetration of single spermatozoa to the ovum may, however, involve the action of sperm-borne enzyme. Although a capacity for new synthesis by sperm seems unlikely, the sperm as a source of the enzyme is well established (394). It would accordingly appear possible that hyaluronidase inhibitors might act as inhibitors of fertility. As indicated in the introduction (page 6), our experience with several such inhibitors derived synthetically from hyaluronic acid was that an antifertility effect could be obtained by admixture with sperm suspensions [23 (Ch. 1)] or by intravaginal instillation preceding coitus, but not on parenteral administration. Others appear to have had similar experiences [e.g., Parkes (395) with trigentisic acid]. Our notion was that the materials of rather large molecular weight with which we were dealing probably could not penetrate to the site of fertilization in sufficient (or any) quantity. This might apply to other large molecular weight antihyaluronidases, e.g., the naturally occurring serum factor (396) and certain synthetic polymers (397), but a number of low molecular weight inhibitors have been found active against the enzyme (394), and they, or suitable derivatives, should be investigated as possible inhibitors of fertilization. It is unfortunate that the claim for oral antifertility action of phosphorylated hesperedin, a hyaluronidase inhibitor (398), has not been substantiated (399, 400). Similarly, some indications that hyaluronidase added to rabbit sperm suspensions might increase fertility (391) could not be confirmed (401). The net result has been a perhaps premature abandonment of research on hyaluronidase in relation to fertility. The recent demonstration of the antifertility effect by oral administration to male rats of ammonium aurine tricarboxylate, a hyaluronidase inhibitor, may revive interest. Since there was no effect of this compound on sperm morphology or motility, Schoysman and Wesel (392) conclude that sperm penetration of either cervical mucus or of the ovum was prevented. This should be readily ascertainable experimentally.

Austin (373) has discussed possible chemotactic substances concerned with sperm attraction to ova. Direct evidence for such substances in mammals is rather tenuous. Most suggestive is the tendency in mice for sperm bearing the *t* allele to fertilize preferentially ova carrying the same allele (402). Whether this accounts for the superiority in fertilization of sperm of one strain over another in mixed inseminations of rabbits (403) and in certain mouse genotypes (404) or whether modified agglutinin effects are involved requires further study.

Mention should be made here of a seminal constituent that may affect the tubal transport of ova. This is the vasodepressor first described by von Euler (405) and called prostaglandin. It has recently been found to have a specific effect on the Fallopian tube, increasing the tonus and contraction amplitude maximum in the proximal part with a reverse effect on the rest of the tube (406). This should lead to retention of the ova in the middle part of the tube, thus facilitating fertilization. Its use in excess and its antagonism should be worth observing. Actually several prostaglandins have been isolated and identified chemically (407) and two of them have been found to be identical with the stimulant of myometrium found in menstrual fluid (408). Control of uterine transport of eggs and sperm may be effected by these compounds.

The penetration of the zona pellucida of the egg by sperm appears to occur as the result of the action of a sperm-borne lytic agent. The demonstration of such an agent in the acrosome of invertebrate sperm has been made (401, 409, 410). Austin [9 (Ch. 1)] has presented some evidence for a similar acrosome reaction in mammalian sperm. However, no active lytic agent has been as yet extracted from mammalian sperm, and proteolytic enzymes shown to act on the zona are not demonstrably carried by spermatozoa. Nor has any lytic action of hyaluronidase upon the zona been shown. Nonetheless, as Rothschild (411) has pointed out, a practically universal event occurring at the time of the penetration of the first sperm is a definite change in the nature of the egg membrane(s) initiated at the point of entry and leading to alterations in the physical-chemical properties and generally (depending upon the time taken to completion) to the exclusion of extra spermatozoa. In mammals, this has been called the "Zona reaction" (412). It is possible that the same sperm-borne lysin that effects zonal passage also initiates the zona reaction. For purposes of fertility control, a thorough investigation of natural or contrived factors affecting and including the zona reaction would appear to be worthwhile. Perhaps the most tantalizing barrier to efficient pursuit of this problem is the still highly variable degree of success in effecting fertilization of mammalian eggs in vitro. The firm establishment of a consistent, repeatable in vitro fertilization is from many points of view an outstanding desideratum. Where it has been accomplished in the rabbit with some success the susceptibility to developmental variations has been shown by the effects of an antimetabolic agent (*413*).

Following hyaluronidase action *in vitro* to remove the cumulus of freshly ovulated rabbit ova, Chang and Bedford (*414*) managed by shaking to disperse the corona cells remaining. Such naked ova transferred to insemination-recipient females showed a remarkable reduction in fertilizing capacity. Presumably the adherent cells act as sperm guides or maintainers of fertilizing capacity. The acceleration of guard cell removal *in vivo* may be an experimental possibility. Even more suggestive is the finding that only one of 673 rat ova transferred to the Fallopian tubes of mated rabbits gave evidence of zona penetration by rabbit sperm (*415*). The nature of this barrier to foreign sperm merits further inquiry.

The administration of antibodies against sperm as a means of inhibiting fertilization has been attempted with signal success. Sperm suspensions of one species mixed with antiserum produced in another species may indeed be rendered incapable of fertilization (*416, 417*) but such immune serum administered parenterally apparently cannot inhibit fertilization. It is interesting that an immune serum prepared in cattle against rabbit semen (or rabbit erythrocytes) will, on direct incubation *in vitro* or *in utero,* increase significantly the death rate of 9-day embryos. However, antiserum incubated 1-day ova were not significantly damaged (*418*). Antibodies to bull sperm (but not to rabbit sperm) have been found in rabbit uteri following systemic immunization, but fertilization occurs normally (*419*). Perhaps by adequate analysis to determine the ovum processes affected and the specific antibody doing the job, clues to the causes of this embryo mortality may be had. Now we know only that immunization even to homologous sperm or testis preparation often leads to lowered fertility (*420*). The possibility of autoimmunity so effectively shown by Freund *et al.* (*421*) when they induced aspermatogenesis in guinea pigs with a single injection of homologous testis tissue plus adjuvant has not led to practical outcomes in other species.

Beside the fertilizin-antifertilizin concept, no comprehensive accounting for the "fertilization reaction" has emerged. Studies of ovum metabolism preceding, during, and following fertilization have been made mostly in nonmammalian species. No uniform pattern of metabolism characterizes each of these states. For example, in some species fertilization increases, in others it decreases, and in others it effects no change in respiratory metabolism (*411*). Attempts to find characteristic reactants in or products of fertilization have had some success in a given species, but no universally occurring fertilization substances have been found. The few studies of the metabolism of mammalian ova have been confined practically exclusively to postfertilization stages since the presence of actively metabolizing follicle cells about the unfertilized eggs and also during fertilization offers an insuperable obstacle to measurements of ovum-specific processes by the usual *in vitro* techniques.

TABLE 13
SPERM SURVIVAL TIMES IN THE FEMALE TRACT[a]

Animal	Maximal duration of fertility (hr)	Maximal duration of motility (hr)	Reference
Rabbit	30–32	—	*422*
Mouse	6	13	*423*
Guinea pig	21–22	41	*424, 425*
Rat	14	17	*426*
Ferret	36–48	—	*84* (Ch. 2)
Sheep	30–48	48	*427, 428*
Cow	28–50	—	*429, 430*
Horse	144	144	*431, 432*
Man	28–48	48–60	*56* (Ch. 2), *433, 434*
Bat	135 days	159 days	*435*

[a] From Bishop [*51* (Ch. 2)].

Although the biochemical events occurring in mammalian eggs at fertilization are essentially unknown, the fate of eggs and sperm as fertilizing agents has been the subject of extensive inquiry. Establishment of the duration of fertility has been sought for a number of mammalian species. In Table 13, taken from Bishop [*51* (Ch. 2)], it is clear that for the most part maintenance of fertilizing capacity by sperm in the female reproductive tract is measured in hours. In the horse, demonstrable fertility has been retained for some days, and, in the bat, sperm inseminated in the fall maintain fertility through hibernation and into the spring. Measures which might reduce or protract the duration of sperm-fertilizing capacity have not been examined to any great extent experimentally. The inhibition of uterine sperm capacitation by progesterone administration [82 (Ch. 2)] may involve an adverse effect on the duration of sperm-fertilizing capacity; and a search for the intrauterine factor(s) involved is most desirable. Similarly, the thus-far unidentified factor(s) in seminal plasma which inhibit sperm capacitation (369) should be identified. Intrauterine spermatotoxins [30 (Ch. 1)] act as agents to separate sperm heads from tails, as direct lethal agents, and perhaps as inciters to sperm phagocytosis. In addition, substances toxic to mature sperm and ordinarily examined *in vitro* or by administration to males (e.g., ethyleneimino compounds or sulfonoxy alkanes) should be administered to females having sperm *in utero*. The recent demonstration that visible radiation kills avian and mammalian sperm (436) *in vitro* suggests not light *in utero*, but further study of the photoreceptive pigment responsible. The action of ionizing radiation on sperm, of course, has been extensively studied. In mammals, sublethal doses may lead to gynogenesis, a condition that never eventuates into viable embryos (437). This suggests a possible role for radiomimetic agents.

Mammalian ova also have a limited fertilizable life. This is illustrated in Table 14, taken from Blandau [89 (Ch. 2)]. Again, this is a matter of hours, and there is some variation from species to species. The possible bases of this limited fertilizable life have also received little attention. That the ambient temperature is a highly significant factor has been beautifully demonstrated by Chang (452) who showed that brief exposures of unfertilized rabbit ova to high temperatures would inhibit fertilizability, whereas storage at lower temperatures would maintain fertilizability for several days. This is illustrated in Fig. 6 which suggests that anything which is hyperthermic (e.g., pyrogens) might be fertility-inhibiting. In an experimental study in the rabbit, Chang [83 (Ch. 2)] found that a 3–4 hour fever due to administered pyrogen did not affect early ovum development, but faulty implantation and fetal development did occur. Other factors which might affect the duration of fertilizability of ova may be rather diverse, *i.e.*, they may involve endogenous conditions that exert autolytic or cytolytic action upon ova, there may be a slow, spontaneous (enzymatic?) development of the zona reaction or the vitelline sperm-blocking reaction, there may be a hormone-conditioned tubal milieu which becomes adverse in the luteal phase. The observation that progesterone administration inhibits fertilization in the rabbit [78 (Ch. 2)] and that norethynodrel will accomplish this in the rat [234 (Ch. 4)] may be

TABLE 14

THE FERTILIZABLE LIFE OF THE MAMMALIAN OVUM[a]

Animal	Length of fertilizable life	Investigator	Ref.
Opossum	Morphologic signs of degeneration appear within 24 hr after ovulation	Hartman, 1924	(439)
Mouse	(a) 12 hr, Matings 13 hr after ovulation result in reduced fertility	Long, 1912	(440)
	(b) 6 hr, estimation	Lewis and Wright, 1935	(441)
	(c) 8 hr, experimental	Runner and Palm, 1953	(442)
Hamster	5 hr, experimental	Chang and Fernandez-Cano, 1958	[83 (Ch. 2)]
Rat	>12 hr, experimental	Blandau and Jordan, 1941	(443)
Guinea pig	>20 hr, experimental	Blandau and Young, 1939; Rowlands, 1957	(444) (445)
Ferret	>30 hr, experimental	Hammond and Walton, 1934	[83 (Ch. 2)]
Rabbit	6 hr, experimental	Hammond, 1934	(446)
	8 hr, experimental	Chang, 1953	[8 (Ch. 1)]
		Braden, 1952	(447)
Sheep	24 hr, estimation	Green and Winters, 1935	(448)
Cow	18–20 hr, experimental	Barrett, 1948	(449)
Mare	Short	Day, 1940	(450)
Monkey	23 hr, estimation	Lewis and Hartman, 1941	(451)
Man	6–24 hr, estimation	Hartman, 1936	[85 (Ch. 2)]

[a] From Blandau [89 (Ch. 2)].

explained as a rendering of the eggs unfertilizable by a progestin-labile reaction in the Fallopian tubes. It is clear that ovicidal agents acting upon the unfertilized eggs are conspicuously unknown. If unfertilized ova exhibited a special susceptibility to irradiation, one might turn to likely irradiation-induced organic peroxides. Unfortunately, unfertilized rabbit and hamster ova are rather remarkably radiation resistant (453). Clues to agents which might act to

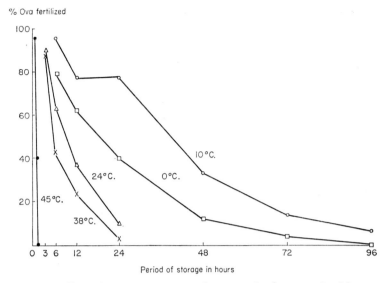

FIG. 6. Effect of temperatures on subsequent fertilization of rabbit ova. [From Chang (*452*).]

prolong the life of unfertilized eggs are even more scant. However, it is tempting to question why it is that ova maintained within the ovary for many years as viable entities lose their vitality in a matter of hours when they are liberated from the follicle.

REFERENCES

364. Pincus, G., and Enzmann, E. V. 1953. *J. Exptl. Med.* **62**, 655.
365. Moricard, R., and Gothie, S. 1953. In "Mammalian Germ Cells" (G. E. W. Wolstenholme, ed.), p. 180. Little, Brown, Boston, Massachusetts.
366. Mattner, P. E. 1963. *Nature* **199**, 772.
367. Chang, M. C. 1959. *Nature* **184**, 466.
368. Venge, O. 1953. In "Mammalian Germ Cells" (G. E. W. Wolstenholme, ed.), p. 243. Little, Brown, Boston, Massachusetts.
369. Chang, M. C. 1957. *Nature* **179**, 258.
370. Austin, C. R. 1963. *J. Reprod. Fertility* **6**, 313.
371. Bently, R. A., and Mukherjee, D. P. 1963. *J. Reprod. Fertility* **6**, 261.
372. Bedford, J. M. 1963. *J. Reprod. Fertility* **6**, 245.
373. Austin, C. R. 1963. In "Mechanisms Concerned with Conception" (C. G. Hartman, ed.), p. 285. Macmillan, New York.
374. Lillie, F. R. 1919. "Problems of Fertilization." Univ. of Chicago Press, Chicago, Illinois.

375. Tyler, A. 1959. *Exptl. Cell Res.* Suppl. 7, 183.
376. Bishop, D. W., and Tyler, A. 1956. *J. Exptl. Zool.* 132, 575.
377. Thibault, C., and Dauzier, L. 1960. *Compt. Rend. Acad. Sci.* 250, 1358.
378. Thibault, C., and Dauzier, L. 1961. *Ann. Biol. Anim. Biochim. Biophys.* 1, 277.
379. Chalmel, M. 1962. *Ann. Biol. Anim. Biochim. Biophys.* 2, 279.
380. Kalwaryjski, B. E. 1926. *Biochem. Z.* 169, 355.
381. Lindahl, P. E., and Nilsson, A. 1954. *Arkiv Zool.* 7, 223.
382. Lindahl, P. E. 1960. *J. Reprod. Fertility* 1, 3.
383. Lindahl, P. E. 1959. *Exptl. Cell Res.* 16, 394.
384. Pincus, G., and Enzmann, V. E. 1936. *J. Exptl. Zool.* 73, 195.
385. Austin, C. R. 1948. *Nature* 162, 534.
386. Blandau, R. J., and Odor, D. L. 1949. *Anat. Record* 103, 93.
387. Braden, A. W. H., and Austin, C. R. 1954. *Australian J. Biol. Sci.* 7, 543.
388. Moricard, R., and Bossu, J. 1951. *Fertility Sterility* 2, 260.
389. Chang, M. C. 1951. *Ann. Ostet. Ginecol.* (2nd Fasc. Spec.) p. 918.
390. Braden, A. W. H. 1953. *Australian J. Biol. Sci.* 6, 693.
391. Chang, M. C. 1950. *Ann. N. Y. Acad. Sci.* 52, 1192.
392. Schoysman, R., and Wesel, S. 1962. *Compt. Rend. Soc. Biol.* 156, 1701.
393. Odor, D. L., and Blandau, R. J. 1951. *Am. J. Anat.* 89, 29.
394. Meyer, R. K., and Rapport, M. M. 1952. *Advan. Enzymol.* 13, 199.
395. Parkes, A. S. 1953. *Lancet* ii, 285.
396. Glick, D., and Moore, D. H. 1948. *Arch. Biochem.* 19, 173.
397. Hahn, L., and Frank, E. 1953. *Acta Chem. Scand.* 7, 806.
398. Sieve, B. F. 1952. *Science* 116, 373.
399. Chang, M. C., and Pincus, G. 1953. *Science* 117, 274.
400. Millman, N. N., and Rosen, F. 1953. *Science* 118, 212.
401. Tyler, A. 1949. *Am. Naturalist* 83, 195.
402. Braden, A. W. H. 1960. *J. Cell. Comp. Physiol.* 56, 17.
403. Beatty, R. A. 1960. *J. Reprod. Fertility* 1, 52.
404. Braden, A. W. H. 1958. *J. Genet.* 56, 37.
405. von Euler, U. S. 1934. *J. Physiol.* (*London*) 81, 102.
406. Sandberg, F., Ingleman-Sundberg, A., and Ruden, G. 1963. *J. Obst. Gynaecol. Brit. Commonwealth* 70, 130.
407. Bergström, S. 1963. *Biochem. Pharmacol.* 12, 413.
408. Pickles, V. R., and Hall, W. S. 1963. *J. Reprod. Fertility* 6, 315.
409. Colwin, L. H., and Colwin, A. L. 1960. *J. Biophys. Biochem. Cytol.* 7, 315.
410. Colwin, A. L., and Colwin, L. H. 1960. *J. Biophys. Biochem. Cytol.* 7, 321.
411. Rothschild, Lord V. 1956. "Fertilization." Methuen, London.
412. Braden, A. W. H., Austin, C. R., and David, H. A. 1954. *Australian J. Biol. Sci.* 7, 391.

413. Bomsel-Helmreich, O., and Thibault, C. 1962. *Ann. Biol. Anim. Biochim. Biophys.* **2,** 265.
414. Chang, M. C., and Bedford, J. M. 1962. *Fertility Sterility* **13,** 421.
415. Dickmann, Z. 1962. *J. Reprod. Fertility* **4,** 121.
416. Parsons, E. I., and Hyde, R. R. 1940. *Am. J. Hyg.* **B31,** 89.
417. Kiddy, C. A., Stone, W. H., and Casida, L. E. 1959. *J. Immunol.* **82,** 125.
418. Menge, A. C., Kiddy, C. A., Stone, W. H., and Casida, L. E. 1962. *J. Reprod. Fertility* **4,** 87.
419. Edwards, R. G. 1960. *J. Reprod. Fertility* **1,** 385.
420. Katsh, S. 1959. *Am. J. Obst. Gynecol.* **77,** 946.
421. Freund, J., Lipton, M. M., and Thompson, G. E. 1953. *Bull. N. Y. Acad. Med.* **29,** 739.
422. Hammond, J., and Asdell, S. A. 1926. *J. Exptl. Biol.* **4,** 155.
423. Merton, H. 1939. *Proc. Roy. Soc. Edinburgh* **59,** 207.
424. Yochem, D. E. 1929. *Biol. Bull.* **56,** 274.
425. Soderwall, A. L., and Young, W. C. 1940. *Anat. Record* **78,** 19.
426. Soderwall, A. L., and Blandau, R. J. 1941. *J. Exptl. Zool.* **88,** 55.
427. Green, W. W. 1947. *Am. J. Vet. Res.* **8,** 299.
428. Dauzier, L., and Winterberger, S. 1962. *Ann. Inst. Rech. Agron. No. 1,* 13.
429. Laing, J. A. 1945. *J. Agr. Sci.* **35,** 72.
430. Vandeplassche, M., and Paredis, F. 1948. *Nature* **162,** 813.
431. Day, F. T. 1942. *J. Agr. Sci.* **32,** 108.
432. Burkhardt, J. 1949. *J. Agr. Sci.* **39,** 201.
433. Rubenstein, B. B., Strauss, H., Lazarus, M. L., and Hankin, H. 1951. *Fertility Sterility* **2,** 15.
434. Horne, H. W., Jr., and Audet, C. 1958. *Obstet. Gynecol.* **11,** 421.
435. Wimsatt, W. A. 1942. *Anat. Record* **83,** 299.
436. Norman, C., Goldberg, E., and Porterfield, I. D. 1962. *J. Exptl. Cell Res.* **28,** 69.
437. Beatty, R. A. 1964. "International Symposium on Effects of Ionizing Radiation on the Reproductive System," p. 229. Pergamon Press, New York.
438. Chang, M. C. 1956. *Ann. Ostet. Ginecol.* **14,** 74.
439. Hartman, C. G. 1924. *Am. J. Obstet. Gynecol.* **7,** 40.
440. Long, J. A. 1912. *Univ. Calif. (Berkeley) Publ. Zool.* **9,** 105.
441. Lewis, W. H., and Wright, E. S. 1935. *Contrib. Embryol., Carnegie Inst. Washington* **25,** 113.
442. Runner, M. N., and Palm, J. 1953. *J. Exptl. Zool.* **116,** 1.
443. Blandau, R. J., and Jordan, E. S. 1941. *Am. J. Anat.* **68,** 275.
444. Blandau, R. J., and Young, W. C. 1939. *Am. J. Anat.* **64,** 303.
445. Rowlands, I. W. 1957. *J. Endocrinol.* **16,** 98.
446. Hammond, J. 1934. *J. Exptl. Biol.* **11,** 140.

447. Braden, A. W. H. 1952. *Australian J. Sci. Res., Ser. B* **5**, 460.
448. Green, W. W., and Winters, L. M. 1935. *Anat. Record* **61**, 457.
449. Barrett, G. R. 1948. "Time of Insemination and Conception Rates in Dairy Cows." Ph.D. Thesis, University of Wisconsin, Madison, Wisconsin.
450. Day, F. T. 1940. *J. Agr. Sci.* **30**, 244.
451. Lewis, W. H., and Hartman, C. G. 1941. *Contrib. Embryol., Carnegie Inst. Washington* **29**, 1.
452. Chang, M. C. 1952. *J. Exptl. Zool.* **121**, 351.
453. Harvey, E. B., and Chang, M. C. 1962. *J. Cell. Comp. Physiol.* **59**, 293

CHAPTER 6

Free Ovum Development

We have just remarked on the limited duration of fertilizability of mammalian ova. Unless fertilization occurs degeneration soon sets in and the signs are unmistakable. Visibly the egg cytoplasm will fragment, shrink, crinkle; the chromosomes depart from the spindle and scatter or clump or resolve into irregular or numerous subnuclei. In contrast, the act of sperm penetration vitalizes the ovum; the deliquescence of senility is averted and there ensues the vital succession of pronucleus formation and orientation, syngamy, mitosis, and first cleavage. Fertilization is, however, not a complete insurance to vitality. In the rat, for example, about 10% of ovulated ova fail to implant in the uterus [24 (Ch. 1), 454] and this is due in part to the failure of fertilized ova to develop normally. A small percentage may be polyspermic eggs in which the presence of the extra sperm has blocked cleavage or has induced a triploid condition which may survive through a few divisions (455), but which does not appear to be compatible with full fetal development (459).

Polyspermy appears to occur with considerable frequency when fertilization occurs late after ovulation. As much as 50% of pig ova from late inseminations will give evidence of polyspermy (456, 457). Trinucleate eggs so formed or those formed as the result of failure of second polary body extrusion (458), which has been shown to occur in late matings in the golden hamster [83 (Ch. 2)], appear to have no chance for survival. Also, hyperthermy may increase polyspermy (455), but any significant natural occurrence of this is dubious.

103

Probably the cleaving egg leads a relatively untroubled existence in its slow progression through the Fallopian tube into the uterus. According to the best evidence at present available, fertilization normally takes place at the junction of the tubal ampulla and isthmus. In the rabbit, the cumulus mass surrounding the egg takes from 4½ to 12½ minutes to reach this junction where it then remains for at least one hour (459). Thereafter the eggs progress quite slowly through the relatively short isthmus, taking about 3 days to reach the uterus. In most mammals this isthmus passage lasts for 3 to 3½ days, but in the ferret, the dog, and the cat stays of 5 days or longer have been reported, and in the opossum and wallaby only 24 hours [89 (Ch. 2), 460].

In Table 15 are presented the approximate times to the development of various cleavage stages, blastocyst development, uterine entry, and implantation. The physiological bases for the variations in the rate of development and duration of these early stages in the free ova are far from elucidated. Endogenous growth-limiting factors probably exist as Hartman has shown for the opossum (462). Indeed, sperm may contribute mutagen-induced dominant genes lethal or sublethal to the cleaving ovum (463). But the access of essential nutritive factors, special vascular conditions, and hormonal variations are some of the significant exogenous factors.

Indeed, the major regulatory influence on the tubal transport of eggs appears to be ovarian hormone. The contrasting responses of the tubal musculature, the ciliary beat, and even the secretory cells to estrogen and progestin have been detailed by numerous investigators [see 89 (Ch. 2)]. Very briefly summarized, in the follicular phase of the cycle or on estrogen administration tubular contractions tend to be of large amplitude and relatively infrequent, ciliary movement tends to speed up and the tubal fluid is produced in increased amount. In contrast, in the luteal phase of the cycle, or on progesterone administration, the contractions are of much less amplitude and more frequent, peristalsis is less violent, ciliary movement is lessened and fluid secretion reduced. One would expect, therefore, that any hormonal influence upsetting the normal sequence from the follicular to the luteal phase of ovarian activity would also alter the fate of the cleaving ova in the Fallopian tubes. Experimentally this was first demonstrated in mice and rabbits receiving moderate doses of estrogen during postfertilization days [*18* (Ch. 1), *464, 465*]. Two effects were noted: (a) a retention of the ova in the Fallopian tubes (tube locking) long past the time they would normally enter the uterus and (b) an eventual degeneration of the cleaving ova. In contrast, massive doses of estrogen administered to rats and mice accelerated the passage of ova through the Fallopian tubes and the uterus with consequent sterility (*466, 467*). These sterilizing effects of estrogen administration

TABLE 15

APPROXIMATE CLEAVAGE RATES AND TUBAL TRANSPORT
AND IMPLANTATION TIMES[a]

Animal	2-Cell	4-Cell	16-Cell	Blastocyst	Entry into uterus (days)	Implantation
Man[b]				5–8 days	3	8–13 days
Rat[c]	1–2 days	2–3 days	4 days	4½ days	3	5–6 days
Mouse[c]	21–23 hr	38–50 hr	60–70 hr	66–82 hr	1.45	4–5 days
Rabbit[c]	21–25 hr	25–32 hr	40–47 hr	75–96 hr	2.5–4	7–8 days
Guinea pig[c]	23–48 hr	30–75 hr	107 hr	115 hr	3.5	6 days
Monkey[b]	26–49 hr	24–52 hr	4–6 days		3	9–11 days
Horse	24 hr	30–36 hr	98–100 hr		4	8–9 weeks
Cow[b]	27–42 hr	50–83 hr	4 days	8–9 days	3–4	30–35 days
Sheep[c]	38–39 hr	42 hr	3 days	6–7 days	2–4	17–18 days
Pig[c]	25–51 hr	25–74 hr		5–6 days	3–4	11 days
Ferret[c]	51–71 hr	64–74 hr	95–120 hr	4½–6 days	5–6	7–8 days
Mink[c]	3 days	3–4 days	5–6 days		8	25 days
Cat[c]	40–50 hr	3 days	4 days	5–6 days	4–8	13–14 days

[a] From data recorded principally by Beatty (*459*).
[b] Times from ovulation.
[c] Times from coitus (first coitus with mink).

have been observed in several species and with the use of both synthetic and natural estrogens (*468, 469, 471*). In the mouse, testosterone administration also causes tube locking and sterility (*470*), presumably by similar effects on the musculature of the tubouterine junction. In the rat, progesterone administration accelerates the passage of tubal ova [*94* (Ch. 2)].

We shall return to a more detailed discussion of ovum transport, but here it should be stressed that there is no simple rule relating the action of hormonal steroids or hormonally active nonsteroidal agents to tubal responses. Thus Greenwald (471) has found that estradiol cyclopentylpropionate administered to rabbits at low doses accelerates tubal passage of ova and at high doses causes retention. Again, norethynodrel, which is an oral gestagen in the rabbit, will also induce the expulsion of tubal ova in the rabbit, but it may also cause tubal retention of some ova (472). Clomiphene, an anti-estrogen, accelerates ovum passage in rabbits (472) and rats (473).

The ovarian hormones affect not only tubal musculature but also the secretory activity of the Fallopian tubes. This has been elegantly demonstrated in recent years by Mastroianni and his colleagues who have developed a technique for the quantitation of tubal secretions in the conscious rabbit and rat (474, 475). Castration causes a marked decrease in tubal fluid secretion; this may be restored by estrogen administration. Progesterone inhibits the estrogen effect in castrate females as well as in normal, estrous rabbits. Indeed, Mastroianni et al. (476) have demonstrated that the anti-estrogen, 1-(p-2-diethylaminoethoxyphenyl)-1-phenyl-2-p-anisylethanol, known as MER-25, significantly decreases tubal secretion in both intact rabbits and estrogen-primed castrates. In estrogen-treated rats, the depressant effect observed within 24 hours following a single injection of MER-25 is followed by a return to pre-injection levels.

The reduction in tubal secretion caused by MER-25 may be responsible for the degeneration of tubal ova that occurs following its oral administration [90 (Ch. 2), 477]; however a direct effect on the cleaving ova in vitro has been demonstrated (478, 479). Similarly another anti-estrogen, a derivative of 2,3-diphenylindene (U-1155A) appears to act as an antifertility agent in laboratory mammals only during the period of ovum cleavage (480). Direct ovicidal effect is not excluded here either since a number of other anti-estrogens administered during late cleavage inhibit implantation in rats and mice in a manner entirely similar to that obtained by estrogen administration (481). Indeed, Jolley et al. (482) have demonstrated a direct inhibition of sea urchin egg cleavage by estradiol added to the medium. The rather high inhibiting concentration $(3 \times 10^{-3} M)$ is certainly not attained in mammalian Fallopian tubes *in vivo* even with exogenous estrogen administration. It should be noted at this point that not all anti-estrogens are anti-fertility agents. Those which have been most studied for this property such as MER-25, U-1155A, and the anti-estrogens of the stilbestrol series (483) are nonsteroidal. A large number of steroidal anti-estrogens are known. The prototype is progesterone, and practically all of the synthetic progestins are, by standard assay, estrogen inhibitors (484, 485). As progestins, these compounds ordinarily favor ovum development and implantation. Furthermore, their progestational potency and anti-estrogenic potency are usually parallel (486). The standard tests for anti-estrogenic activity involve inhibition of estrogen-induced growth changes in the rodent vagina or uterus. By these criteria, MER-25 is a rather poor anti-estrogen, whereas dimethylstilbestrol and 17-ethynyl-19-nortestosterone are excellent inhibitors (481, 482). In turn, MER-25 does not inhibit estrogen action on the pituitary whereas the progestins do (487).

Direct effects upon cleaving ova have been obtained with a number of antimitotic agents. The ovicidal effect appears to be accomplished without any effects upon the hormonal balance of the mother. The antimitotic agents *d*-usnic acid and podophyllotoxin have been found to be especially potent in rats (488). In the rabbit, Adams *et al.* [101 (Ch. 2)] have observed a lethal effect on cleaving ova of administered 6-mercaptopurine, 8-azaguanine, triethylenethiophosphoramide (Thio TEPA), β-bis-1,6-chloroethyl-amino-D-mannitol (Degranol), triethylenemelamine (TEM), *N*-desacetyl-*N*-methylcolchicine (Colcemid), and *N*-desacetylthiolcolchicine (Thiolcolceran). A direct mitosis-inhibiting effect of colchicine on fertilized rabbit ova culture *in vitro* has long been known (489). Culture of rabbit ova *in vitro* with the antibiotics penicillin, Chloromycetin, paromomycin, and penicillin-G may, at relatively high concentrations, result in prevention of development on transfer to recipients (490), but no *in vivo* effects of antibiotics have been reported.

From the foregoing evidence, it is clear that the cleaving tubal ova may be manipulated experimentally by two major methods: (a) altering hormonal influences on the Fallopian tubes and (b) direct action of mitosis-affecting agents. Nonetheless, your author is left with a definite feeling of dissatisfaction at this point. This is probably due to a hiatus between the inducing cause and the observed end result. If a tubal nutrition is indeed altered by estrogens or anti-estrogens, are specific constituents of tubal secretion involved? By what mechanism is the rate of tubal secretion altered? In the case of the mitosis-inhibiting agents, we presumably are fairly close to an action upon the energy-producing mechanisms of the cleaving ovum. We have a rather meager knowledge of these energy-producing systems and how they operate in mammalian eggs. One generalization can be made: All mammalian eggs thus far studied decrease in mass during cleavage. Hamilton and Laing (491) have calculated the decreases as follows: sheep, 40%; ferret, 30%; mouse, 25%; cow, 20%. Presumably the utilization of the storage material or deutoplasm is involved. Our knowledge of the chemical nature of mammalian deutoplasm is negligible. We do know that in the rabbit ova it contains oxidizable substrate in sufficient concentration to sustain oxygen uptake at a rate which is not significantly altered by pre-incubation, nor by the presence of substrate in the medium [91 (Ch. 2)]. Since glucose as the energy source in the cleaving egg is metabolized practically exclusively via the hexose monophosphate oxidation pathway and glycolysis appears to be negligible [92 (Ch. 2)], the cleaving egg should have special sensitivity to inhibitors of pentose and TPNH (triphosphopyridine nucleotide, reduced form) production. Presumably the pentose makes a major contribution to nucleic acid synthesis and the TPNH to reductive processes involved in lipid synthesis. These presumptions are open to experimental verification and may offer a firm biochemical basis for assaults on the cleaving egg.

A potent means for the study of cleavage dynamics is offered by the fact, previously noted, that the ova of some species may cleave *in vitro* at approximately normal rates. Thus mouse ova may be carried to the blastocyst stage in a fairly simple culture medium, a Krebs-Ringer bicarbonate solution with added lactate and bovine albumin (492, 493). Golden hamster ova, which may be successfully fertilized *in vitro*, still fail to exhibit more than a single cleavage in a variety of test media (494). Sooner or later many species will yield to *in vitro* ovum cleavages with consequent multiple opportunities for experimental manipulation.

REFERENCES

454. Pincus, G. 1956. *Acta Endocrinol. Suppl.* **28**, 18.
455. Austin, C. R., and Braden, A. W. H. 1953. *Australian J. Biol. Sci.* **6**, 674.
456. Pitkojenen, I. K. 1955. *Izv. Akad. Nauk S.S.S.R* **3**, 120.
457. Hancock, J. L. 1959. *Animal. Prod.* **1**, 103.
458. Thibault, C. 1959. *Ann. Zootech. Suppl.* **8**, 165.
459. Beatty, R. A. 1957. "Parthenogenesis and Polyploidy in Mammalian Development." Cambridge Univ. Press, London and New York.
460. Harper, M. J. K. 1961. *J. Reprod. Fertility* **2**, 522.
461. Austin, C. R. 1959. *In* "Reproduction in Domestic Animals" (H. H. Cole, and P. T. Cupps, eds.), Vol. I, p. 339. Academic Press, New York.
462. Hartman, C. G. 1953. *In* "Mammalian Germ Cells" (G. E. W. Wolstenholme, ed.), p. 253. Churchill, London.
463. Partington, M., and Jackson, H. 1963. *Genet. Res.* **4**, 333.
464. Burdick, H. O., and Pincus, G. 1935. *Am. J. Physiol.* **111**, 201.
465. Burdick, H. O., Whitney, R., and Pincus, G. 1937. *Anat. Record* **67**, 513.
466. Burdick, H. O., and Whitney, R. 1937. *Endocrinology* **21**, 637.
467. Whitney, R., and Burdick, H. O. 1937. *Endocrinology* **22**, 639.
468. Parkes, A. S., Dodds, E. C., and Noble, R. L. 1938. *Brit. Med. J.* **II**, 557.
469. Velardo, J. T., Raney, N. M., Smith, B. G., and Sturgis, S. H. 1956. *Fertility Sterility* **7**, 301.
470. Burdick, H. O., Emmerson, B. B., and Whitney, R. 1940. *Endocrinology* **26**, 1081.
471. Greenwald, G. S. 1963. *J. Endocrinology* **26**, 133.
472. Chang, M. C. 1964. *Fertility Sterility* **15**, 97.
473. Davidson, O. W., Schuchner, E., and Wada, K. 1964. *Anat. Record* **148**, 274.
474. Mastroianni, L., Jr., and Wallach, R. C. 1961. *Am. J. Physiol.* **200**, 815.
475. Mastroianni, L., Jr., Beer, F., Shah, U., and Clewe, T. H. 1961. *Endocrinology* **68**, 92.
476. Mastroianni, L., Jr., Abdul-Karim, R., Shah, U., and Segal, S. J. 1961. *Endocrinology* **69**, 396.
477. Chang, M. C. 1959. *Endocrinology* **65**, 339.
478. Segal, S. J., and Tyler, A. 1958. *Biol. Bull.* **115**, 364.
479. Chang, M. C. 1964. Personal communication.
480. Duncan, G. W., Stucki, J. C., Lyster, S. C., and Lednicer, D. 1962. *Proc. Soc. Exptl. Biol. Med.* **109**, 163.
481. Emmens, C. W., and Finn, C. A. 1962. *J. Reprod. Fertility* **3**, 239.
482. Jolley, W. B., Martin, M. E., Bamberger, J. W., and Stearns, L. W. 1962. *J. Endocrinol.* **25**, 183.
483. Emmens, C. W., Cox, R. I., and Martin, L. 1959. *J. Endocrinol.* **18**, 372.
484. Edgren, R. A. 1958. *Endocrinology* **62**, 689.
485. Dorfman, R. I., Kincl, F. A., and Ringold, H. J. 1961. *Endocrinology* **68**, 17.
486. Edgren, R. A. 1961. *Nature* **190**, 353.

487. Culter, A., Ober, W. B., Epstein, J. A., and Kupperman, H. S. 1961. *Endocrinology* **69**, 473.

488. Wiesner, B. P., and Yudkin, J. 1955. *Nature* **176**, 249.

489. Pincus, G., and Waddinton, C. W. 1939. *J. Heredity* **30**, 515.

490. Hafez, E. S. E. 1962. *Fertility Sterility* **13**, 583.

491. Hamilton, W. J., and Laing, J. A. 1946. *J. Anat.* **80**, 194.

492. Brinster, R. L. 1963. *Exptl. Cell Res.* **32**, 205.

493. Gwatkin, R. B. L. 1963. *Proc. Natl. Acad. Sci. U. S.* **50**, 576.

494. Yanagimachi, R., and Chang, M. C. 1964. *J. Exptl. Zool.* **156**, 361.

CHAPTER 7

Blastocyst Development
and Implantation

In Chapter 2 we indicated that the entry of the ovum into the uterus is marked by: (a) significant alterations in endogenous development and metabolism and (b) an environment markedly conditioned by regulatory hormones and definitely limiting ovum nutrition. That the uterine environment is not *essential* for ovum growth and development has been demonstrated by their culture *in vitro*, their continued growth in extra-uterine environments, and, in some species, by ectopic pregnancy. Mouse (*495, 496*) and rabbit (*497*) ova that have been transplanted to the anterior chamber of the eye show normal cleavage, but failure of development occurs later. Transplantation beneath the kidney capsule of rat (*498*) and mouse (*499*) ova generally leads to survival with varying degrees of embryo development, depending upon the stage at the time of transfer. Transplantation of mouse blastocysts into the spleen leads usually to luxuriant trophoblast growth with rare embryo differentiation (*500*). Reciprocal transplants of cleaved ova between mice and rats, on the other hand, are marked by normal development to implantation stages, but failure of decidual evocation (*501*). Similarly, sheep or cattle ova in rabbit uteri develop normally for about 5 days from cleavage to late blastocyst stages (*502, 503*). Thus it may be said that an uterine environment tends to evoke *normal* development to implantation stages, but further normality is had only if nidation occurs. We have already demonstrated the remarkable dependence of the implantation process on a properly progestin-conditioned uterus. That the inadequate uterus may indeed act as a positive inhibitor of the blastocyst as a nidating organism is rather startlingly suggested by Lutwak-Mann *et al.* (*504*) who found that blastocysts recovered from rabbits ovariectomized 17–26 hours previously were incapable of implantation although they would grow apparently normally in culture and on transfer *in vivo*. It is almost as if the spayed rabbit's uterus produces an implantation inhibitor that is stored up by the blastocysts. Similarly, Kirby (*505*) has shown that mouse ova forced to remain (by ligation) in the Fallopian tubes for more than 3½ days although normal in appearance will not implant on transfer to the uterus, suggesting a tubal antagonistic factor at a critical time.

The act of implantation itself is rigidly conditioned. Chang (*506*) was the first to demonstrate in the rabbit that unless transplanted blastocysts were within one day of the host uterus in developmental age implantation would not occur. Dickman and Noyes (*507*) extended these observations to the rat and found that transferred ova one day younger than the cornua would degenerate on the fifth day. Ova one day older than the cornua would delay their development until the uterine development attained functional synchronization; then normal blastocyst implantation would occur. Long survival in the uterus in a state of arrested development is an event occurring naturally in some species and is contrivable experimentally in others. Delay of implantation for as long as 10 months has been claimed for the badger, 9 months in the fisher, 6 months in bears and the American badger, 4 months in the European roe deer, and so on [*89* (Ch. 2), *508*]. In the rat, mouse, and several insectivores, lactation concurrent with ovum development leads to delay of implantation. In the rodents we have shown that the length of this delay is proportional to the number of young sucking (*509*), and presumably the hormonally conditioned ovum growth-promoting factor of the uterus is in abeyance during the period of delay (*510*).

Regardless of the latent period to implantation the blastocyst at the time of nidation appears to be a guided organism. First of all in any given species a characteristic method of attachment to the endometrium must operate; for example the macaque blastocyst attaches to both walls of the uterus and remains within the lumen, but the chimpanzee blastocyst migrates through the uterine epithelium, lodges in the stroma, and becomes covered in by epithelium. The macaque thus forms an epithelial plaque and the characteristic stromal decidual reaction does not occur (*511, 512*). Second, the spacing of the blastocyst appears to occur in a fairly determined sequence. In the rabbit, for example, during the first 2 days in the uterus the ova appear to distribute at random, but thereafter a spacing mechanism appears to operate to insure even distribution (*511*). That ovarian hormones act upon blastocyst distribution has been clearly shown by the behavior of ova transplanted to control and estrogen-treated, ovariectomized rabbits (*513*). Finally, evidence for more than passive participation in the "moment of implantation" is the finding that casting off of the remnants of the zona pellucida depends upon blastocyst, not uterine, action at a limited time (*514*).

Ovarian Hormones and Implantation Processes

The hormone dependence of implantation time in most mammals is emphasized by experimental alteration in the period of uterine survival and the time of implantation. In rats ovariectomized on the second day after mating, subliminal doses of progesterone (0.5 mg/day) will maintain the ova for as long as 45 days, and implantation may be induced by increasing the progesterone dose or by administering a very small dose of estrogen (*515*). Blastocysts in rats ovariectomized on the fourth day will survive *in utero* for 3 weeks or longer, but progesterone alone can no longer induce implantation; estrogen is necessary along with progesterone (*516–518*). In the rat the exact timing of ovariectomy may markedly affect progesterone-induced implantation. Thus Zeilmaker (*519*) finds progesterone administration will sustain implantation in rats ovariectomized at the first hour on day 4, but not in those ovariectomized 8 hours previously. In a similar way prolactin will maintain ovum implantation in rats hypophysectomized at the seventeenth hour of day 3, but not in animals hypophysectomized 3 hours earlier. The latter effect may involve the pituitary-induced estrogen surge occurring at day 3 to 4 in the rat (cf. 540). Psychoyos (520) finds implantation in rats may be delayed by trifluoperazine (the tranquilizer Stelazine) administered from day 3 on; this delay is overcome by concomitant estradiol administration indicating replacement of the missing surge of estrogen. Zeilmaker (519), however, found no inhibition of implantation by either atropine sulfate or reserpine administered on day 3, although a reduced size of implantation sites was noted. Since the induction of implantation in rats ovariectomized before or during day 4 requires both estrogen and progesterone (521), Nutting and Meyer (522) have used the day 3 ovariectomized rat as a test animal for the effectiveness of various synthetic gestagens as the progesterone substitute in maintaining blastocyst viability. 17α-Ethyl-19-nortestosterone proved to be 6.4 times and 21-fluoro-17-acetoxyprogesterone or 6α-methyl-17-acetoxyprogesterone 47.5 times as active as progesterone. Neither testosterone propionate, norethylnodrel, nor ethynodiol diacetate were active while 17α-ethynyl-19-nortestosterone was weakly active at 1 mg but not at 4 mg doses. Just as the lowest dose of estrone leading to prompt implantation also leads to maximal embryo survival (523), so were the lower effective doses of the progestins optimal for postimplantation survival.

In contrast to the rat, implantation in the armadillo will occur in the absence of hormone replacement (524). The possibility of another source of progestin and estrogen has not been excluded, i.e., the adrenal cortex. However, in the armadillo, excision of corpora lutea alone invariably prevents implantation, suggesting a positive anti-implantation factor (perhaps estrogen) in the ovary (525). In rats ovariectomized and adrenalectomized on day 4, estrogen and progesterone will effectively induce implantation (517); corticosterone will not substitute for the estrogen (526). In the hamster castrated on day 2 progesterone acts only in appropriate dose to normal implantation, never to delay (527); indeed in this species testosterone allegedly acts as a progestin synergizing with estrogen (528).

It is clear from the foregoing that implantation depends upon progestin-estrogen regulated series of events involving both the receptor tissue and the ovum. What is this series of events? May it be defined with some exactitude? On the basis of morphological data available for the critical period, Blandau [89 (Ch. 2)] finds species differences of such a nature that a general theory of implantation seems unlikely. Shelesnyak, on the other hand, has amassed a body of experimental data chiefly with the rat that has led to the formulation of just such a general theory (529, 530). The evocation of the decidual reaction of the uterine endometrium is apparently the key phenomenon (Fig. 7). Blandau points out

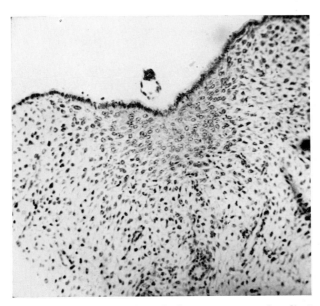

FIG. 7. Longitudinal section through the antimesometrial wall of a pregnant rat killed on the fifth day. The loosely attached rat blastocyst has initiated the subepithelial decidual response. There is no detectable alteration in the superficial epithelium. ×450 [51 (Ch. 2)].

that this is evoked in certain species, e.g., the rat, the bat, by slight mechanical pressure such as that given by glass or paraffin beads inserted into the uterus. In other species, e.g., the guinea pig, monkey, and man, where the reaction normally is initiated by embryo removal of the superficial epithelium, a certain amount of trauma or damage is necessary; glass or paraffin beads will not evoke the decidual reaction in the guinea pig (531). Thus, depending upon the species, mechanical pressure alone or tissue damage presumably due to lytic enzyme action may lead to the basic reaction essential to implantation. Böving (532) believes that trophoblast invasion in the latter case involves a negative feedback system in which the stimulative substance enters the maternal circulation and stimulates the regulatory hormone system to react upon the endometrium. Shelesnyak claims that histamine is the responsible active substance for the initiation of the decidual reaction (529). It may arise subtly at a pressure point or more obviously from damaged mast cells.

Basic to the Shelesnyak hypothesis is the notion of an "estrogen surge" into a progestin-conditioned uterus without which surge nidation cannot occur. That estrogen evokes increased histamine concentration in the rat uterus has been demonstrated by Spaziani and Szego (533), and by deduction the estrogen surge also yields a histamine increase. Thus the administration of an active antiestrogen (MER-25) on the day of the surge inhibits nidation in rats bearing blastocysts and the formation of decidua ordinarily formed following a single intraperitoneal injection of pyrathiazine hydrochloride (534). The pyrathiazine is an antihistaminic which causes histamine release (535). Estrogen in a single dose administered to rats ovariectomized preceding the surge tended to restore decidualization capacity (534). Histamine antagonists (536) or agents markedly depleting the histamine supply (537) tend to interfere with both nidation and the decidual reaction. Studies of uterine metabolism indicate marked increases during pyrathiazine-induced decidualization in the concentrations of protein, DNA, and RNA. A peak in these uterine concentrations in pseudopregnancy occurs on days 4 and 5, presumably consequent on the estrogen surge. Ethanoxytriphetal inhibits both the pseudopregnant peak and the decidual rise (538).

In attempts to repeat these experiments, Orsini (539) found pyrathiazine relatively ineffective as a deciduomagenic agent in the rat and hamster, and she concluded that genetic factors might account for the differences in the rats used. In the progestin-estrogen sensitized rabbit, Chambon (540) finds that histamine in any dose employed fails to evoke deciduoma (see also 541). Some trauma is needed as well. Indeed Chambon concludes that a complex of endometrial factors are involved, not the least of which may be acetylcholine release. Banik and Ketchel (542), finding trauma deciduomagenic in one uterine horn of pregnant and pseudopregnant rats and finding histamine, even in large doses, ineffective in the other horn, conclude that histamine release is an effect and not a cause of deciduomagenic activity. Finn and Emmens (543) have found that in pseudopregnant rats the frequency of occurrence of deciduoma formed after cervical stimulation may be markedly reduced by the administration of dimethylstilbestrol, a potent anti-estrogen. However, estradiol in $\frac{1}{80}$ the dose also reduces deciduoma frequency. It has long been known that excess estrogen will inhibit the deciduoma reaction (544), and Emmens, recognizing that dimethylstilbestrol is a proestrogen as well as an anti-estrogen, wonders if its effect may not be due to conversion in adequate amount to an estrogen. Ethanoxytriphetal is not an estrogen or proestrogen by conventional assay but since it does have a weak uterotropic action (545) it may mimic estrogen as an antideciduomagen. Emmens (546) alleging possible estrogenic contaminants in histamine samples even suggests that histamine-induced deciduoma may be a low-dose estrogen phenomenon and that intrauterine antihistamines may be merely toxic to uterine tissue and not functionally suppressive. The inability of systemically administered antihistaminics to suppress decidualization or nidation (547, 548) has been attributed by Shelesnyak (536) to their rapid detoxification and poor intrauterine concentration. The demonstration by Glenister (549) of rabbit blastocyst implantation into endometrial explants in organ culture offers a means for direct study of implantation processes and perhaps some answers to the present somewhat controversial situation.

Extra-ovarian Influences on Implantation

That hormonal influences other than the ovarian play a role in implantation processes is suggested by findings such as those of Kar and Sen (550) who demonstrated an increase in the number of implantations in thyroid hormone treated rats. More interesting perhaps is the demonstration by Fernandez-Cano (551) that in rats the stresses of high temperature and hypoxia inhibit implantation, presumably by some adrenal secretory product since adrenalectomy suppressed the effect. That an effect on the ovaries via the alarmed pituitary is indeed unlikely is suggested by the finding that ACTH-stimulating stress does not increase LH secretion in the rat (552). Although exogenous corticosteroids may affect fetal growth (553), even quite large doses fail to sterilize mice or rabbits (554). Curiously, in these last experiments 95% of the offspring of prednisolone-treated mice and 66% of the rabbit young were sterile. Both ACTH and cortisone have interrupted pregnancy in the rabbit and the rat (555).

In contrast, triparanol, which upon administration to pregnant rats causes prolonged gestation, multiple cases of fetal resorption, and stillbirths, has no such effect if ACTH is administered simultaneously (556). Presumably its inhibition of cholesterologenesis either leads to inadequate corticosteroid production or to abnormal antifertility adrenocortical products.

Serotonin, which may affect implantation indirectly by reducing progestin secretion, will inhibit deciduoma formation directly in mice (557). Furthermore, its implantation-inhibiting action may be counteracted by an antagonist, methylsergide, as well as by progesterone. A second antagonist, aryoheptadine, inhibits the effects on placental circulation but acts alone as an implantation inhibitor and can be counteracted by progesterone administration (558).

Although the histamine hypothesis of implantation has involved much study of this biologically active amine, the possible role of other biologically important substances in this important intrauterine event has not been completely neglected. The concentrations of certain vitamins, salts, other inorganic substances, sugars, and enzymes have been measured in the uteri of various species during pregnancy [81 (Ch. 2), 559]. Some of the variations have been interpreted as functional to implantation and pregnancy maintenance. Outstanding is the remarkable increase during early pregnancy or pseudopregnancy of endometrial carbonic anhydrase in the rabbit, originally described by Lutwak-Mann [237 (Ch. 4)]. As can be seen in Fig. 8, the peak concentration is reached at the eighth day and then declines (560). In the rat, uterine β-glucoronidase concentration increases to a maximum on day 4 and is maintained to implantation (561). In the rabbit, the endometrial secretions and mucosa on day 6, just preceding implantation, contain appreciable amounts of ATPase, 5-nucleotidase, and purine nucleosidase (562). Changes in activities attributable to a number of other endometrial enzymes characterize pseudopregnancy and early pregnancy; these vary from estrogen-dependent dehydrogenases (563) and β-glucuronidase (564) to a peptidase activity

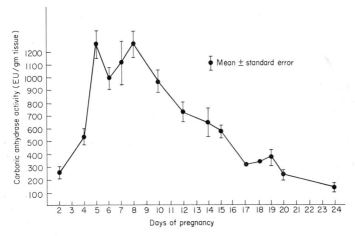

Fig. 8. Carbonic anhydrase activity of endometria from pregnant rabbits (560).

peaking at the time of implantation (565). The possible functional significance of each change has been reviewed by Hafez (566). Inositol has been found in rabbit uterine fluids and its concentration is particularly influenced by progesterone (567). Similarly, an increase in uterine fluid bicarbonate to twice that of the plasma has suggested the active secretion of the ion by the endometrium (568).

Lutwak-Mann (559) has compared the concentrations of certain constituents in rabbit blastocysts with their concentrations in the maternal blood serum. Her data are presented in Table 16. The free, 6-day blastocysts are relatively poor in total nitrogen, total phosphorus, and glucose, but have high concentrations of potassium and especially of bicarbonate. Even the implanted blastocyst at day 8 exhibits a relatively low content of nitrogen and phosphorus, but potassium and bicarbonate have fallen to maternal levels. The association of high bicarbonate with the blastocyst (and uterine fluid) at implantation time has led Böving to a hypothesis which states that progestin-stimulated uterine carbonic anhydrase facilitates bicarbonate transfer from the blastocyst and that the attendant local liberation of alkalinity makes both the membranes

TABLE 16

CHEMICAL COMPOSITION OF RABBIT BLASTOCYST AT
IMPLANTATION STAGE AT GESTATION[a]

Constituents	Concentration	Age from time of mating (days)		
		6[b]	7	8
Total nitrogen	mg/100 gm	30–35	40–78	300–420 (845)[c]
Total phosphorus	mg/100 gm	2.0–2.5	2.8–3.2	4.2–5.0 (10.4)
Sodium	meq/liter	137–139	118–126	128–145 (150)
Potassium	meq/liter	10–12	10–14	4.5–6.5 (7.1)
Chloride	meq/liter	71–74	70–76	78–89 (106)
Total reducing sugar	mg/100 gm	3–10	46–68	66–77 (100)
"True" glucose	mg/100 gm	—	42	62 (85)
Bicarbonate	μl CO_2/ml	1500	800–1100	480–500 (520)

[a] From Lutwak-Mann (559).
[b] Entire blastocysts were used at 6 days; at 7 and 8 days the blastocyst fluid was withdrawn by aspiration.
[c] Values in parentheses refer to analyses in maternal blood serum.

and the trophoblast sticky and thus initiative of attachment (532, 569). He is not unmindful, however, of the fact that in other species carbonic anhydrase is not a conspicuous constituent of the endometrium during the luteal phase. Indeed, in the mouse uterus it is estrogen which increases carbonic anhydrase, and this effect is antagonized by progestin (560, 570, 571). Most engaging is Boving's comment: "Also warning against assuming carbonic anhydrase to be absolutely essential rather than merely normally present and helpful, is its absence from the endometrium of many species other than the rabbit. This variation introduces the fascinating idea that implantation in different mammals differs in fundamental chemistry just as it differs endocrinologically and anatomically."

The blastocysts' development of a degree of dependence on the maternal circulation following implantation indicates that barriers to possible toxic agents may exist in the endometrium or in the ovum itself. The fact that the blastocyst fails to implant but continues to develop in rabbits ovariectomized on day 6 just before normal implantation time (504) makes it possible to determine that the free 7-day blastocyst has the same glucose and bicarbonate content as the implanted ovum, but a lower lactic acid content. Cortisone-induced hyperglycemia in rabbits is counteracted by stilbestrol, but these effects are seen in the implanted, not in the free, blastocyst (572). Salicylates penetrate directly to the free blastocysts from the endometrium, but do not affect ovum metabolism.

The Lability of Implantation Processes

Without wishing to alarm the reader, I give you in Table 17 the scheme for the study of ovum implantation evolved in 1959 by Eckstein, Shelesnyak, and Amoroso (573). This is the encyclopedic approach which says let us know everything from every point of view, and then perhaps we'll understand. Nonetheless, implantation is a process occurring at a critical time under delicately balanced conditions in an organism and in its special environment. To the analytically minded, the delineation of the mechanism of such a process may be attained by seizing on one or more of its cardinal attributes and reducing it (or them) to their basic events. For reasons both theoretical and practical, an inquiry into the lability of the implantation process to various inhibitory agents may repay the inquiring mind. Let us consider, therefore, the various means whereby implantation may be inhibited and the significance of these means for the control of fertility.

Returning to the fundamental situation, we have a living, developing organism, the blastocyst, receiving nutrition in an intrau-

TABLE 17

SCHEME FOR STUDY OF OVUM IMPLANTATION[a]

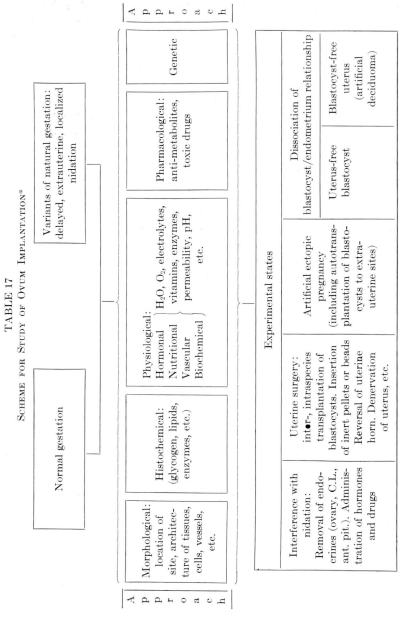

Normal gestation			Variants of natural gestation: delayed, extrauterine, localized nidation

Approach

Morphological: location of site, architecture of tissues, cells, vessels, etc.	Histochemical: (glycogen, lipids, enzymes, etc.)	Physiological: Hormonal, Nutritional, Vascular, Biochemical } H_2O, O_2, electrolytes, vitamins, enzymes, permeability, pH, etc.	Pharmacological: anti-metabolites, toxic drugs	Genetic

Experimental states

Interference with nidation: Removal of endocrines (ovary, C.L., ant. pit.). Administration of hormones and drugs	Uterine surgery: inter-, intraspecies transplantation of blastocysts. Insertion of inert pellets or beads Reversal of uterine horn. Denervation of uterus, etc.	Artificial ectopic pregnancy (including autotransplantation of blastocysts to extrauterine sites)	Dissociation of blastocyst/endometrium relationship	
			Uterus-free blastocyst	Blastocyst-free uterus (artificial deciduoma)

[a] From Eckstein et al. (573).

terine environment which is maintained as adequately, but not excessively, growth-promoting to the blastocyst by a balanced action of estrogen and progestin primarily upon the endometrium. One means of disequilibrating such a balanced state is to have an excess of any one of its constituents. An excess of blastocysts may be achieved by superovulation and mating. This has indeed been examined experimentally in rabbits (574), sheep (575), and mice (576, 577). Reduced fertility and fecundity is the rule, due apparently to two factors: (a) the failure of implantation in a large proportion of the animals [e.g., 50% of the mice in experiments of Wilson and Edwards (577)] and (b) mortality of fetuses in the overcrowded uterus and often difficult parturition with a degree of maternal mortality. The latter (b) may be overcome by careful husbandry of the superovulated animals, but the former (a) may represent an effect of ovarian hormone imbalance since all superovulating treatments stimulate ovarian steroid secretion (578, 579), perhaps with an excess of certain constituents over others, at least for a limited time. No one who has seen the remarkably hypertrophied ovaries of the superovulated cow with their numerous corpora lutea can fail to be impressed with the suggested potency for hypersecretion (Fig. 9). Actually in superovulated mated heifers, a premature entry of fertilized ova into the uterus has been recorded (580), and in superovulated rabbits accelerated passage has also been reported (581).

Estrogens and Anti-estrogens

This premature expulsion of the ova from the Fallopian tubes has recently been demonstrated in estrogen-injected rats (582), rabbits (583), and guinea pigs (584, 585). Estradiol cyclopentylproprionate was administered in a single injection on the first postcoital day to rats, and the uteri were examined for embryos on the eleventh day. On the basis of the corpora lutea formed 19, 66, and 95% of the expected embryos were missing with doses of 1, 5, and 10 μg, respectively. Further study indicated that decidua formation could be induced in the first two groups but not in the 10 μg recipients. Furthermore, practically all ova were expelled through the uterus by 48 hours postcoitum. Using the same tech-

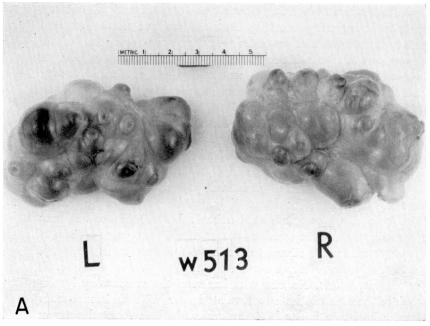

FIG. 9. A. Ovaries from beef cattle after superovulation by gonadotropins, 3000 IU of PMS followed by 2000 IU of HCG 5 days later. Note the developing corpora lutea. The cow was slaughtered 5 days after the HCG injection. B. Superovulated ovary from a 3-month-old calf treated with 3000 IU of PMS followed by 300 IU of HCG 5 days later; 146 ovulation points were counted. Note the size of ovaries compared with the immature uterus. From Hafez (*580*).

nique of injection of estradiol cyclopentylproprionate on day 1 in rabbits, the same investigator found 86, 97, 100, and 100% of embryo deaths by day 8 with 25, 50, 100 and 250 μg doses, respectively. Here at the lowest dose embryo expulsion from the uterus occurred in 48 hours, but an endometrium with normal pseudopregnant proliferation was observed on day 8. At the high estrogen dose, tube locking of the ova occurred at the ampullary isthmic junction and blastocyst degeneration was visible by day 5.

In the guinea pig, estradiol benzoate in 5–20 μg doses injected on day one caused accelerated tubal transport and premature expulsion of the eggs from the uterus. When the estrogen in 30–50 μg

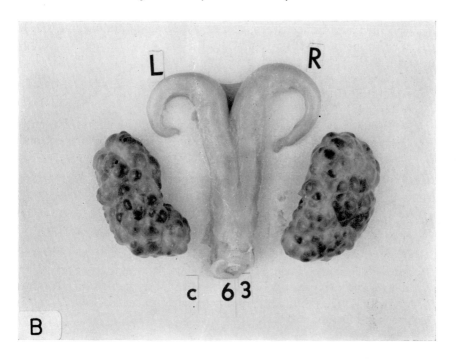

dose was injected after the ova entered the uterus, expulsion did
not occur and implantation took place; postimplantation abortion
was observed in these animals due to suppression of luteal function.
Even ovariectomy on day 5 with estrogen (20 μg) injections on
days 6 and 7 did not inhibit implantation. Thus the apparent inhibition of implantation in the animals receiving estrogen on day one
is really an expulsion of ova (or tube locking) and not an effect on
the endometrial reception mechanism. This may explain the findings
of Edgren and Shipley that estrone administered to the rat on
days 2 and 3 at 40 μg in a single injection will inhibit pregnancy,
whereas a dose of 160 μg administered on day 7 or day 10 is
ineffective (587). The estrogen effect is only partially overcome
in the rat by the simultaneous administration of progesterone
(585). In the mouse, the interruption of early pregnancy by estrogen is not prevented by progesterone or the synthetic progestins
17-ethyl- and 17-ethynyl-19-nortestosterone, nor by 19-nortestos-
terone, although these same compounds will act as anti-estrogens

in other target effects, e.g., uterine hypertrophy and edema (588). Furthermore, 17-ethyl-19-nortestosterone, an effective progestin, will inhibit the antideciduomagenic action of estradiol in rats, but the anti-estrogen ethanoxytriphetal is only slightly inhibitory of the estrogen effect at low dose and at high dose it acts just like estradiol (589).

Emmens and his co-workers have pursued the notion that anti-estrogens might be effective inhibitors of ovum development and implantation. After studying a variety of stilbestrol analogs [483 (Ch. 6)], they found that by several tests dimethylstilbestrol (DMS) was much the most potent inhibitor of estrogen action. In rabbits, its injection at a 25 mg dose on days 5 to 7 led to a 50% failure of implantation (590). Injected into rats and mice on day 4, this compound and various chemical relatives prevented implantation, as did estradiol [481 (Ch. 6)]. In a careful study of stilbestrol analogs in mice, Martin et al. (591) found a remarkable parallelism between their postcoital antifertility, anti-estrogenic and proestrogenic potencies (all of these compounds are metabolized to estrogens in vivo and are therefore proestrogens). In Table 18, I present

TABLE 18

RELATIVE POTENCIES OF ANTIFERTILITY AGENTS OF THE STILBESTROL SERIES[a]

Compound	Antifertility	Anti-estrogenic	Pro-estrogenic
Ethylstilbestrol	0.51 (0.51)[b]	0.87	0.28
Propylstilbestrol	0.40 (0.60)[b]	0.77	0.79
Racemic-butestrol	3.9	1.1	1.1
Meso-butestrol	28.7	8.0	10.3

[a] From Martin et al. (591).
[b] Duplicate assays.

a résumé of their data in which the relative potencies are expressed in terms of DMS as the standard. Because of their proestrogenic potencies, the possibility exists that their effects are due to an estrogen excess rather than to intrauterine inhibition of endogenous estrogen action. Since the action of DMS and estradiol in implantation and deciduoma inhibition is additive in mice, Stone and Emmens (592) again conclude that DMS acts as an estrogen.

In the stilbene series, Emmens et al. (593) find that the dihydroxy alkanes are weak anti-estrogens in mice, and that they fail to interfere with early pregnancy at fairly high dose. Phloretin, which like ethanoxytriphetal, is both a weak estrogen and an anti-estrogen decreases postcoital fertility in rats. But since it is also antigonadotropic in the parabiotic rat assay, a possible effect on the ovary is not excluded (594). We have already described the implantation-inhibiting effect of ethanoxytriphetal. That it is an effective anti-estrogen is clearly seen in its inhibition of estrogen-stimulated uterine growth and alkaline phosphatase in rats (545, 595) and carbonic anhydrase in mice (560). Nonetheless, it may be in the same class as DMS and phloretin, i.e., basically estrogenic in its action.

Another interesting group of nonsteroidal anti-estrogens are derivatives of diphenylindenes and diphenyldihydronaphthalenes. The former have been reported effective fertility inhibitors in rats when administered early in pregnancy and to have presumably a rather specific effect since they are nonandrogenic, nonprogestational, not antigonadotropic and weakly uterotropic (596). Apparently in rats the effect is as inhibitors of blastocyst implantation, but in the hamster they do not interfere with blastocyst function (597). The diphenyldihydronaphthalene derivatives are more stable and more potent than the indene compounds and are orally active in rats, rabbits, and guinea pigs, but not in hamsters, presumably as implantation-inhibiting anti-estrogens (598, 599). Nelson *et al.* (600) have confirmed the special antizygotic effect of these compounds administered on days 1 to 4 of rat pregnancy, and have seen a similar effect with clomiphene (MRL-41). Action against ova delayed in implantation also occurs, suggesting direct action on the ova. Ovum expulsion is not, however, ruled out, and the ineffectiveness against later blastocysts may be a matter of dosage.

m-Xylohydroquinone has been alleged to be an implantation inhibitor by Sanyal (601). A detailed study by Prahlad and Kar (602) has failed to demonstrate this. Chang [472 (Ch. 6)] has compared in the postcoital rabbit the antifertility effects of two nonsteroidal agents, clomiphene and triethylamine, with norethynodrel and two of its derivatives (SC-6091 and SC-11 800); the steroids were more consistently inhibitory of implantation.

Just as estrogen excess will prevent by one means or another the implantation of ova, so will progestin excess be deleterious. Progesterone, administered before mating to rats induced to ovulate with gonadotropin injection, will prevent the implantation that would otherwise have occurred (603). Administered before implantation to castrate rats carrying fertilized eggs, progesterone accelerates the ovum passage and expulsion [94 (Ch. 2)]. When the ovariectomy is performed at the time of uterine entry and progesterone is administered, implantation is prevented (604). In pregnant mink, various progestin-estrogen combinations effectively sterilize, presumably by implantation inhibition (605). Large doses of the synthetic progestin, norethynodrel, will inhibit implantation when administered postcoitally to the rat [201 (Ch. 3), 606]. However, this compound fails to maintain pregnancy in the rat and rabbit, as does its homolog, norethindrone (607). Norethindrone (17α-ethynyl-19-nortestosterone) will inhibit implantation in rats, mice, and rabbits [481 (Ch. 6), 590], but in none of these will the closely related 17α-ethyl-19-nortestosterone act as an inhibitor even in large dose, and in test spayed rats and mice the latter compound will maintain pregnancy (607). The synthetic progestational steroid, DL-13β-ethyl-17β-hydroxy-17α-ethyl-4-gonen-3-one(WY 3475), has the interesting property of inhibiting implantation on administration early in pregnancy in rats, but will maintain pregnancy when given to females spayed after implantation. It is a weak anti-estrogen and may, therefore, before implantation behave like MER-25, an inhibitor of the "estrogen surge" (608).

Antiprogestins

We have sought steroidal inhibitors of implantation by examining a variety of compounds for their antiprogestational effect. A convenient animal for progesterone assay is the estrogen-primed, immature rabbit, the uterus of which responds to progesterone administration by endometrial pseudopregnant proliferation (609). Quantitation of the endometrial carbonic anhydrase in such animals offers a rapid and accurate progestin bioassay [238 (Ch. 4)]. Antiprogestational assay may be accomplished by administering putative progestin inhibitors along with a standard stimulatory dose of progesterone. The antiprogestational effects of four standard estrogens in this type of assay are shown in Fig. 10. Yamashita and Kuronji (*610*) have confirmed the data of Fig. 10 and found that 17α-ethynylestradiol, hexestrol, and estrone-3-methyl ether are as active as the four compounds of Fig. 10, but that estriol-3-methyl ether is less active.

We then proceeded to test 155 steroid compounds in this assay using 1 mg of progesterone as the standard stimulating dose and

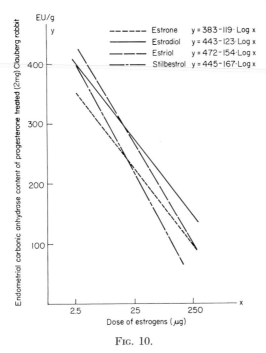

FIG. 10.

emerged with 18 which exhibited significant antiprogestational activity [*95* (Ch. 2)]. These compounds were divisible into two groups, those with two or more double bonds in ring A and those with one or no double bonds in ring A. The structural formulas of the former are presented in Fig. 11 and of the latter in Fig. 12. The compounds of Fig. 11 are estratriene estrogen derivatives (I–X) or neutral steroids having estrogenic activity by ordinary assay and presumably readily metabolized to standard estrogens

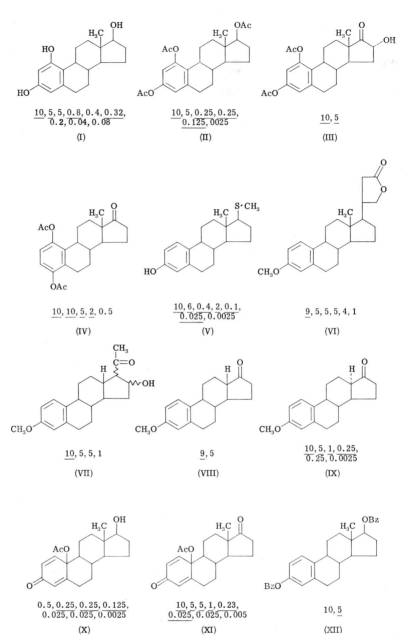

10, 5, 5, 0.8, 0.4, 0.32,
0.2, 0.04, 0.08
(I)

10, 5, 0.25, 0.25,
0.125, 0025
(II)

10, 5
(III)

10, 10, 5, 2, 0.5
(IV)

10, 6, 0.4, 2, 0.1,
0.025, 0.0025
(V)

9, 5, 5, 5, 4, 1
(VI)

10, 5, 5, 1
(VII)

9, 5
(VIII)

10, 5, 1, 0.25,
0.25, 0.0025
(IX)

0.5, 0.25, 0.25, 0.125,
0.025, 0.025, 0.0025
(X)

10, 5, 5, 1, 0.23,
0.025, 0.025, 0.005
(XI)

10, 5
(XII)

Fig. 11. Estrogen derivatives acting as antiprogestins in the rabbit [under-lined doses (mg) are significantly effective].

(XI and XII). Except for the 3-methyl and 3-benzoyl ethers (VI, VII, and X), these active estrogen-like compounds were significant inhibitors at doses well below the standard progesterone dose. We therefore consider these last to be like the standard estrogens of Fig. 10 and designatable as physiological antagonists.

The neutral steroids of Fig. 12, on the other hand, tend to be active at above or at about the standard progesterone dose, and

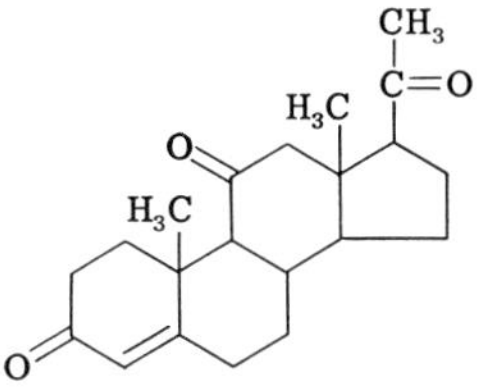

10, 5, 5, 1

(XIII)

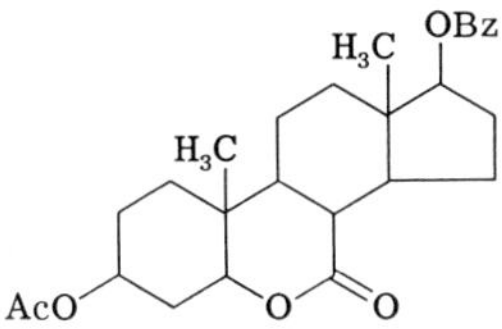

10, 5

(XIV)

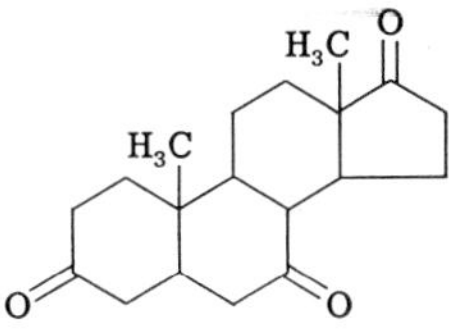

10, 5

(XV)

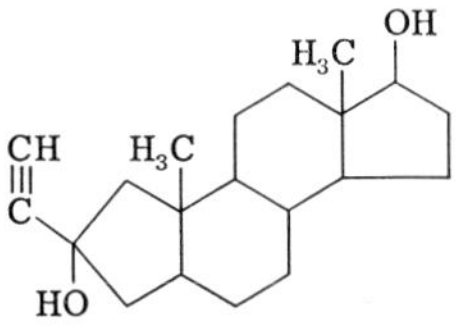

10, 5, 2, 0.5

(XVI)

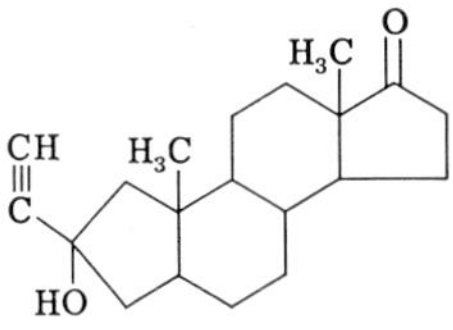

10, 5, 4.0, 0.8

(XVII)

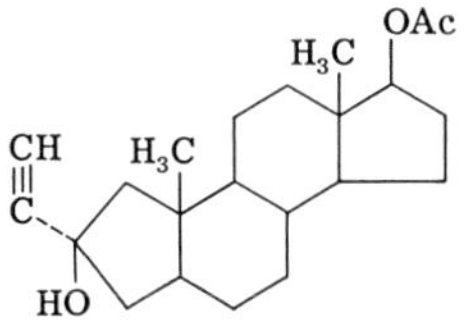

10, 5, 2.5, 1.0, 0.8, 0.4

(XVIII)

Fig. 12. Neutral steroids acting as antiprogestins in the rabbit [underlined doses (mg) are significantly effective].

we thus consider them as probable competitive inhibitors. Yamashita and Kuronji (*611*) have reported that the neutral androgenic steroids 17α-methyltestosterone, androst-4-ene-3,17-dione and androstan-3-ol-17-one are inhibitors at about one tenth the standard progesterone dose. They thus fall somewhat between the active estrogens and the neutral steroids of Fig. 12. The problem of relative potency here is not a simple one since absorption and detoxification rates may differ with the type of compound and thus obscure true potencies at the target site. Furthermore, even in the endometrial tissue itself penetration rates may differ. If, as seems likely, binding to receptor sites is significant for steroid action, then each class of compounds may have specific binding sites and the numbers of such sites may vary widely. Finally, if the steroids affect the rates of either specific separate processes or of linked processes, the velocity coefficient for any given steroid-sensitive reaction may be widely modifiable. We can therefore only classify roughly these antiprogestins on the basis of their relative potencies.

In any event, the notion that antiprogestins should be implantation inhibitors has been put to the test by Dr. Banik and myself (*612*), with rats and mice as the assay animals. Postcoital admin-

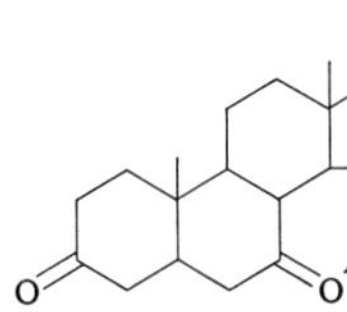

(I)

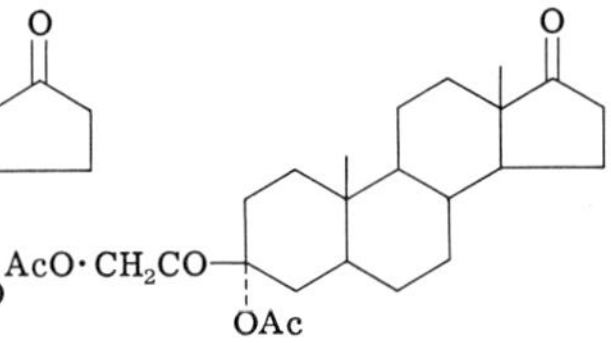

(II)

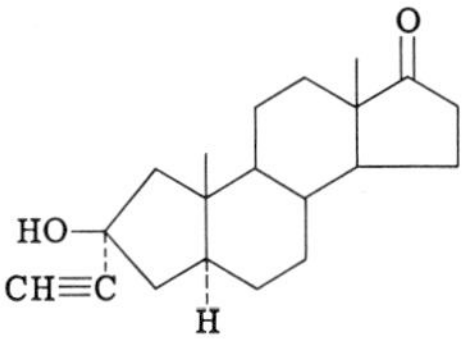

(III)

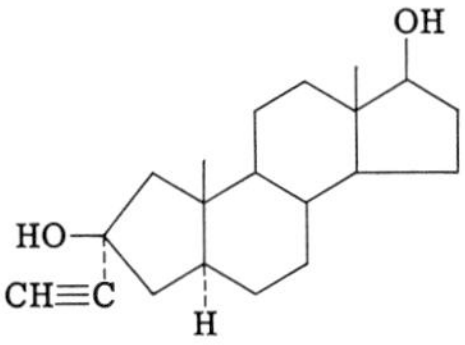

(IV)

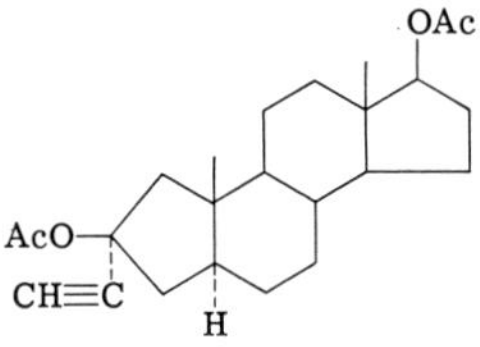

(V)

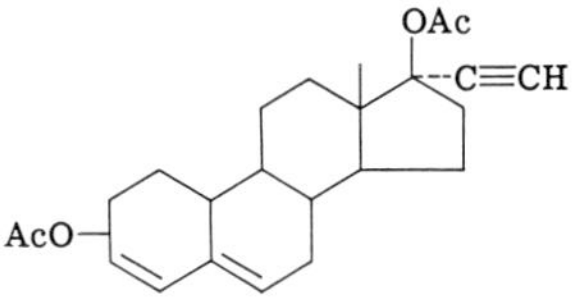

(VI)

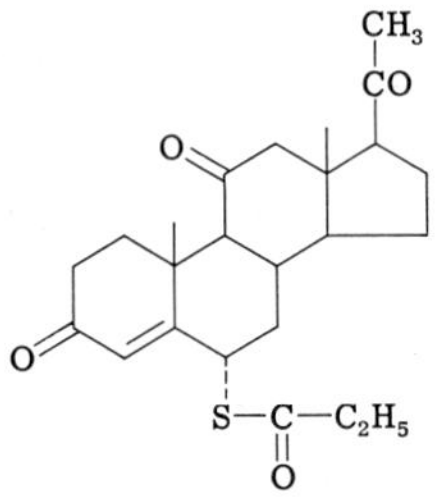

(VII)

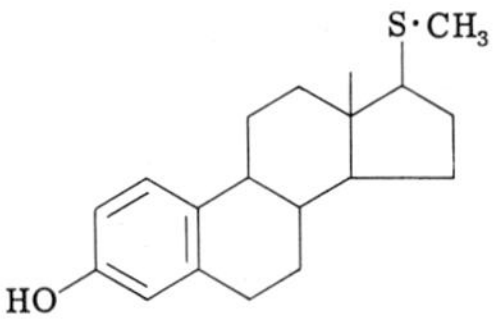

(VIII)

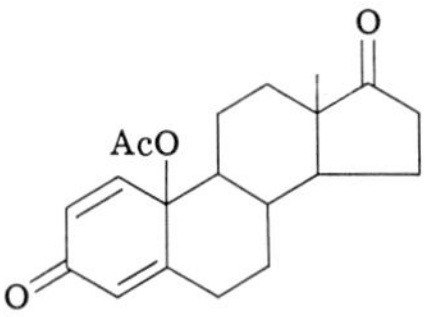

(IX)

FIG. 13. Antiprogestins tested as implantation inhibitors.

istration of the first set of compounds tested was undertaken on days 1, 2, and 3, and implantation was determined on day 11. The formulas of the compounds are presented in Fig. 13. In Table 19 the results of tests of implantation inhibition by the compounds of Fig. 13 are summarized. Several of these (I, II, and VII) are not

TABLE 19

STEROID EFFECTS ON THE IMPLANTATION OF FERTILIZED EGGS
IN RATS AND MICE

Compound number[a]	Animal	Significant implantation-inhibiting dose (mg/day)
I	Rat	None at 2.5 or less
	Mouse	None at 2.5 or less
II	Rat	None at 2.5 or less
	Mouse	None at 2.5 or less
III	Rat	None at 2.5 or less
	Mouse	2.5 but not 0.5
IV	Rat	0.1 but not 0.02
	Mouse	0.02
V	Rat	None at 2.5 or less
	Mouse	0.5
VI	Rat	0.5 but not 0.1
	Mouse	0.1
VII	Rat	None at 2.5 or less
	Mouse	None at 2.5 or less
VIII	Rat	1.0
	Mouse	0.1
IX	Rat	1.0
	Mouse	0.1

[a] The compound numbers refer to those compounds shown in Fig. 13.

active at doses expected to be effective on the basis of their anti-progestational potency. Since the mouse is somewhat more sensitive than the rat, two compounds are found to be active in mice but not in rats (III and V). Finally, four of the nine compounds are clearly active in both species (IV, V, VIII, and IX). We proceeded to examine the potency of these four on injection in a single dose on day 1 and day 3 (Table 20). To our surprise, implantation inhibition was more easily accomplished by administration on day 1 than on day 3. These compounds then resemble the estrogens and anti-estrogens studied by Emmens and his colleagues (*vide supra* page 126). Two of them (VIII and IX) are moderately potent estrogens, having respectively 10 and 3% the activity of estrone in the standard immature mouse uterine weight assay; a third (VI) is both a weak progestin and a very weak estrogen (0.8% of the activity of estrone), and the fourth (IV) is very feebly uterotropic in the immature mouse with an activity approximately $\frac{1}{1500}$ that of estrone. Actually, prevention of implantation may be accomplished with adequate dose on any of the days preceding implantation, but administration after nidation even at fairly high dose is ineffective.

TABLE 20

EFFECTS OF SINGLE INJECTIONS ON OVUM IMPLANTATIONS
IN RATS AND MICE

Compound number[a]	Animal	Significant inhibitory dose (mg) on day	
		One	Three
IV	Rat	1.5	None
	Mouse	0.1	None
VI	Rat	1.0	None
	Mouse	0.1	0.1
VIII	Rat	1.5	None
	Mouse	0.1	?
IX	Rat	1.0	None
		0.1	?

[a] The compound numbers refer to those compounds shown in Fig. 13.

In further tests with chemical relatives of compound IV, the 2,17-diethynyl derivative (X) has proven especially active as an antigestational compound, its minimal effective dose in the rat on administration on day 1 lying between 0.02 and 0.1 mg. On administration for 3 days (1, 2, and 3) 2 μg per day was ineffective but 10 μg significantly effective in blocking implantation. Table 21 gives the data on the effects of single injections on four pre-implantation days compared with a post-implantation day. Obviously, once the embryos are implanted an implantation-inhibiting dose is no longer effective as a sterilizing agent.

We have recently examined a number of other compounds as implantation inhibitors in the postcoital rat and have compared the ratio of this activity (I) to their uterotropic potency in immature mice (U) (*613*). Although compound X proved surprisingly active as a uterotropic agent (about 20% as active as estrone), it was relatively more potent in implantation prevention, giving therefore a ratio U/I of 0.4. Other compounds showed an even more marked separation of these activities, the 17α-difluorovinyl analog of X giving a U/I value of 0.025. Similar separation of antifertility and classic estrogenic effects has been described by Saunders and Rorig (*614*) for several stilbene derivatives. We have tested two of their compounds (*613*) and confirmed this separation.

TABLE 21

Effect of Compound X Injected[a] on Different Dates after Mating upon Pregnancy of Rats

Injection	No. of rats	No. pregnant	P_P	Litter size (Mean ± SE)	P_1
Control	8	7	—	12.85 ± 0.74	—
Day 1	10	1	<0.01	7.0 ± 4.0	<0.05
Day 3	7	0	<0.01	0	Abs. S.[b]
Day 4	7	1	<0.01	7.0 ± 0	<0.05
Day 5	6	0	<0.01	0	Abs. S.[b]
Day 8	6	6	NS[c]	10.83 ± 0.4	NS[c]

[a] One-tenth milligram per rat was injected on different dates after mating. Control animals received vehicle only on day 1.
[b] Absolutely significant.
[c] Not significantly different from control at 5% level.

The relative effectiveness of implantation inhibition by administration in early postcoital days led us to search for the basis of this phenomenon. Two possibilities suggested themselves: (a) an ovicidal effect of the antiprogestin or (b) an effect on the uterine mucosa making it unreceptive to the ova. First of all we studied the movement of fertilized ova in control and compound X-injected rats. The data are presented in Table 22 which shows that in control animals receiving the oily vehicle on day 1 or day 3 practically all of the ova are found at the tubouterine junction. When the usual sterilizing dose was given on day 1 to ten rats, no ova were found in either tubes or uterus on day 4; examination of day-1 injected rats on day 3 disclosed only 3 ova in six rats, and these three were descended into the uterus. Only when ova were collected at 12 hours following compound X administration on day 3 were we able to recover a significant number of eggs, and the majority of these were prematurely descended into the uterus. The ova all appeared healthy and thus their premature expulsion is clearly indicated as the basis for sterilization, resembling the expulsive action of estrogen reported by Greenwald (582) for the rat.

TABLE 22

EFFECT OF COMPOUND X ON MOVEMENT OF FERTILIZED EGGS OF RATS

Treatment	No. rats	No. of blastocysts		
		Fallopian tube	Tubal junction	Uterus
Control: 0.2 ml oil on day 1. Eggs on day 4	6	0	37	0
Control: 0.2 ml oil on day 3. Eggs on day 4	6	0	54	6
0.1 mg on day 1. Eggs on day 4	10	0	0	0
0.1 mg on day 1. Eggs on day 3	6	0	0	3
0.1 mg on day 3, 24 hr before collection	17	0	1	3
0.1 mg on day 3, 12 hr before collection	9	0	9	48

The foregoing data do not prove whether or not any damaging effect is exerted upon the ovum itself. Accordingly, we took ova from normally mated, untreated rats and transferred their ova taken at day 4 to the tubal end of the uteri of recipients made pseudopregnant by mating to vasectomized males on the same day as the fertile mating. Similar transfer of ova was made from rats receiving a sterilizing dose of compound X on day 3½. The number of ova implanted in the recipients was determined on days 10 or 11 and the young delivered at birth were counted and examined. The results shown in Table 23 clearly indicate no ovum damage since 47% of the control ova implanted and 43% of the "treated" and the numbers surviving to birth were also not significantly different. In contrast, we found that 0.1 mg of compound X given on either day 1 or day 5 prevented trauma-stimulated deciduoma formation. Therefore, the antiprogestational action is clearly on the target tissue; not the ova themselves. Compounds IV and X are anti-estrogens by standard assay. The anti-estrogens ethamoxytriphetol and clomiphene also act to prevent implantation when administered during days 1–7 in the rat (*600*). However, they cause embryo death and resorption when administered on

TABLE 23

IMPLANTATION AND DEVELOPMENT OF COMPOUND X-TREATED EGGS[a]

Treatment	No. of eggs transferred	No. implanted	No. pups born	Remarks
Oil control	51	24	20	All pups were found to be in normal shape and good health
0.1 mg/rat on day 3, 12 hr before collection	64	27	23	All pups were found to be in normal shape and good health

[a] All eggs were collected on day 4 of pregnancy of treated animals and transferred to rats on day 4 of pseudopregnancy.

days 8–12 and fail to have an adverse effect (at least at reasonable dose) when given on days 13–17. Curiously this dose, ineffective in mid pregnancy, killed the fetuses on injection on day 18 (*615*).

The antiprogestins used in our study were first identified because of their inhibition of the carbonic anhydrase increase due to progestin action on the rabbit endometrium. In turn, we have studied the effect of non-steroidal carbonic anhydrase inhibitors upon the course of pregnancy in rabbits, rats, and mice. Confirming the work of Adams *et al.* [*101* (Ch. 2)], who found Neptazan which reduced enzyme concentrations markedly in blood and uterus, we have found Diamox and Cardrase to have no effect on systemic administration. However, injected directly into the uterus before implantation, Diamox prevented implantation (*560*), perhaps due to specific blastocyst toxicity.

We have already mentioned that Shelesnyak (*536*) has found certain antihistamines of the ergot series to be deciduoma inhibitors and implantation preventing. In rats, he found ergocryptine to be most effective, ergosine moderately active, and ergocornine practically inactive. Subsequently Carlsen *et al.* (*616*), testing ergocornine methanesulfonate in mice by single subcutaneous injection on days 1–7, found it active only on day 3 or day 4. Shelesnyak and Barnes (*617*) have conducted further experiments with ergocornine in the rat and have indeed found it active, but its action is apparently mediated at at least two levels. The first of these appears to be the hypothalamus where it appears to inhibit luteotropic hormone (LTH) production or release. This locus of action explains its effectiveness despite lack of estrogenic activity on the uterus, its nongonadotropic nature, its inability to affect gonadotropic stimulation of the ovaries. Although its action is reversed by concomitant progesterone administration, the latter merely acts as replacement for inhibited endogenous progesterone. An action via adrenal gland stimulation (or inhibition) has also been disproved. The second level is an unknown tissue locus (perhaps liver) in which the ergocornine is transformed into the active agent. This has been demonstrated by the failure of topical application to ovary, uterus, or hypophysis of pregnant or pseudopregnant rats to affect the course of decidualization or to terminate pregnancy.

Poisons and Antimetabolites

Robson (*618*) has reviewed the action of certain spindle poisons, chromosomal poisons, and antimetabolites upon the course of early and late pregnancy. None of the spindle poisons tested (e.g., trimethyl cochicinic acid methyl ether) significantly affected implantation although they acted adversely on the post-implantation conceptus. The other compounds found to be inhibitors of implantation are listed in Table 24. Most of these drugs are familiar to those interested in cancer chemotherapy studies, and the logic of inhibiting actively dividing embryos by agents affecting tumor growth is obvious. The "therapeutic ratio" of Table 24 is the ratio of the dose causing 100% mortality of the embryos. Clearly DON has the most favorable therapeutic ratio; also its MED is much the lowest, e.g., 2 mg/kg compared with 1000 mg/kg for furazolidine. Methylcholanthrene, a powerful carcinogen, is of interest because it not only is implantation inhibiting but may act as an hormone inhibitor. Jackson and Robson (*619*) have found that its application locally to the target organs antagonizes the effect of the principal sex hormones, estradiol, testosterone, and progesterone, given systemically. Lutwak-Mann and Hay (*620*) have employed the rabbit blastocyst as a test object for the action of similar compounds administered to the mother. In doses nontoxic to the dose 6-mercaptopurine, E-39, thalidomide, and phthaloyl-D-isoglutamine are effective blastocyst poisons.

TABLE 24
COMPOUNDS INHIBITING IMPLANTATION[a]

Compound	Type	"Therapeutic Ratio" in mice
Chlorambucil	Chromosomal poison	2.5
Ethyleneimine benzoquinone (E29)	Chromosomal poison	—
Azaserine	Antimetabolite	—
Thioguanine	Antimetabolite	—
6-Mercaptopurine	Antimetabolite	—
Aminopterin	Antimetabolite	—
6-Diazo-5-oxo-L-norleucine (DON)[b]	Antimetabolite	150
Furazolidine	Antiseptic	2
Methylcholanthrene	Carcinogen	75

[a] From Robson (*618*)
[b] Most active.

The work of Adams *et al.* [*101* (Ch. 2)] suggests differences between the action *in vivo* of various antimetabolites in rabbits. Thus, 6-mercaptopurine and 8-azaguanine cause clear blastocyst degeneration, especially of the embryonic disc. The few embryos that do implant do not survive to term, nor do blastocysts taken from does receiving these compounds and transplanted to uninjected pseudopregnant recipients. Aminopterin is less destructive of blastocysts, and neither 5-bromouracil nor vitamin B_{12} anilide analogs have deleterious effects on the ova. Colcemid, thiolcolciron, thio-TEPA, and triethylenediamine arrest cleavage as well as blastocyst development, whereas Degranol has limited action and Myleran has no antiblastocyst action. The rates of penetration of these compounds into the oviducts may underlie the differences in cytotoxicity; possibly the ovum may have barriers to penetration to some of them. Effects of these and similarly active compounds on ova grown in culture should be illuminating. Studies of rabbit [92 (Ch. 2)] and mouse (621) blastocyst metabolism *in vitro* under the influence of these agents also seem very much in order. Chamberlain (622) has found 6-aminonicotinamide to be a potent inhibitor of implantation in the rat. Joshi *et al.* (623) have reported that cholesteryl chloride appears to inhibit implantation at least partially on administration to young rats. It may act as a cholesterol antagonist in the uterus.

Intrauterine Trauma

Among other attempts to inhibit implantation in experimental animals we should mention intrauterine trauma or pressure devices. Dr. Hafez and I (624) found that the presence of uterine deciduoma prevented implantation of a large proportion of transplanted ova in the rabbit when the age of the ova and the age of the deciduoma were not synchronized. The few ova implanting atrophied soon after. Meyer and Cochrane (625) using the delayed pregnancy device of low dose progesterone to ovariectomized, blastocyst-bearing rats found that deciduoma could be produced by trauma without accompanying blastocyst nidation. The addition of estrogen in low dose induced implantation of the blastocysts despite the presence of the deciduoma. Somewhat less complicated is the finding of Doyle and Margolis (626) that a silk suture placed in the lumen of one horn of a rat's uterus before mating will prevent implantation in that horn after mating. In the nonsutured horn, normal implantation takes place. The sterile horn in this instance contains no deciduoma. In our laboratory Drs. Zipper, Delgado, and Guiloff (627) have studied nylon thread introduction into one horn of rabbits and rats mated 10 days later. In the rabbit, successful implantation, but with abnormal embryo destruction, occurred beyond the immediate area of the thread but never in the area of the thread. In the rat (60 were studied) implantation never occurred in the treated horn as long as the thread was present, but its removal on day 2 allowed some of the blastocysts to implant. Inhibition of progestational development in the area of the thread in the rabbit was evidenced by absence of a decidual reaction and reduction in carbonic anhydrase content, and in the treated horn of the rat by similar lack of decidualization and a rate of isotopic acetate and glucose incorporation into tissue characteristic of the estrous nonpregnant uterus. Other animal experiments with the silver Grafenberg ring in rabbits and monkeys (*628*) and with coiled stainless steel rings in cows (*629*) demonstrated lack of implantation in treated animals. We shall describe some human studies in a later chapter.

Corpus Luteum Inhibition

Mention should be made of the inhibition of implantation in mice by what is called by Parkes the "Bruce Effect" (*630*). This is the finding that 80–90% of newly mated female mice exposed to the proximity of alien males failed to become pregnant and returned to estrus within 7 days as though mating had never taken place. Implantation is prevented in these animals apparently due to failure of corpus luteum maintenance and secretion (*631*). The presence of the alien male is not necessary since placing the females in boxes soiled by males leads to the pregnancy block. Apparently a highly evanescent substance produced by the male acts upon a (hypothalamic) center to inhibit LTH production. This is reminiscent of the effect of ergocornine described above. However, the active substance must be either quite unstable or quite volatile since it cannot be traced to the urine or feces of the males (*632*), whereas a urinary pheromone that advances the time of estrus in mice is demonstrable (*633*).

On the basis of lesion experiments certain limbic brain structures, especially the medial habenula, in the rat appear to be responsible for stimulating LTH production (*634*). A region inhibitory of LTH release seems indicated by the effects of lesions dorsolateral to the paraventricular nucleus made at estrus in cycling female rats (*635*). Prolonged diestrus occurs and uterine deciduoma may be induced. In cows oxytocin administration inhibits the development of corpora lutea and thus induces a precocious estrus (636). The oxytocin-induced lowering of progestin in these corpora lutea may be counteracted by the simultaneous administration of HCG or a crude bovine pituitary extract; neither ovine prolactin, bovine growth hormone nor equine LH are counteractive (637). Oxytocin may therefore repress release of a specific bovine LTH, perhaps acting through a region comparable to that described above for the rat. In pigs, lack of a feedback of progestin on pituitary LTH has been claimed (638) but stilbestrol-induced corpus luteum persistence suggests an estrogen-labile mechanism (639). Corpus luteum regression may be induced in hamsters by estradiol cyclopentylproprionate administration on days 1 or 2 of pregnancy but not when given on day 4. This effect may be counteracted by concomitant administration of PMS, HCG, or ovine FSH but not by prolactin or ovine LH. An estrogen-labile pituitary LTH mechanism is indicated for the first few days of pregnancy or a corpus luteum sustaining action of LH in this species (640). Interference with corpus luteum function by 1α-methyl-allylthiocarbamoyl-2-methyl thiocarbamylhydrazine has been suggested as the basis for implantation prevention and implanted ovum mortality observed in rats consequent on its administration in early pregnancy (641). Similarly the antigonadotropic action of norethynodrel has been held by Saunders (642) to be responsible for its action as a nidation inhibitor on postcoital administration. A double action of this compound is, however, suggested by the finding that at fairly elevated dose it prevents progestin-estrogen sustained nidation in ovariectomized rats (643). The synthetic gestagen medroxyprogesterone acetate (Provera) causes a dosage-dependent delay of implantation in intact rats, which is prevented by the simultaneous administration of a small amount of estrone. Inhibition of endogenous estrogen production by action of the progestin upon pituitary gonadotropin release is held accountable for the implantation delay (644).

An antiserum to sheep LH produced in rabbits has been found to inhibit implantation when injected into rats on days 1–5 of pregnancy (645). This antiserum will suppress estrous cycles in the rat, whereas an antiserum prepared in the same way but with sheep FSH as the antigen had no effect on estrous cycles in the rat (646). Recovery from the effect of the anti-LH antibody occurred in 10 days. The possibility of autoimmunity to LH is the finding of normal estrous cycles, but no ovulation in older hamsters, and/or of immunity to LTH since fertilized ova transplanted to their oviducts fail to proceed to term (647).

Abortion

Many of the procedures which prevent ova from implanting will also cause resorption or abortion of implanted embryos. It is not our purpose to review here the numerous abortion-inducing agents that have been investigated in animal experiments. Robson (618) gives an excellent account of the action of spindle poisons (e.g., TME), chromosomal poisons (e.g., chlorambucil), and anti-metabolites (e.g., DON) pointing out that notable distinctions may be made between direct effects on the fetus and effects following systemic administration. Thiersch has reviewed earlier work [102 (Ch. 2)] and published some of his more recent data on anti-metabolites (648, 649) indicating quite favorable therapeutic ratios for several [e.g., 6-thioguanine, 6-(1-CH$_3$-4'-nitro-5'-imidazolyl) mercaptopurine]. The sterilizing action of 5-hydroxytryptamine may be inhibited in pregnancy in mice by the administration of progesterone or prolactin, but no protective action of these hormones is had late in pregnancy when the drug may kill all fetuses within a half hour (650). An effect on the uterine contents late in pregnancy is therefore indicated. Since its injection into the embryo is not effective whereas injection into the mother is, an effect on the placental vasculature is most likely (651). The interruption of pregnancy in the rat by certain antihistamines seems also to depend on an interference with placental blood flow (652).

The abortion-inducing effects of various natural and synthetic steroids in rats has been reviewed by Marois (653) and of general endocrine agents by Zarrow [81 (Ch. 2)]. Hyperestrinism, a potent cause of sterility in cattle, may be mimicked in its sterilizing aspects by estradiol administration both early and late in pregnancy (654). A rather remarkable abortifacient action of HCG has been observed in the mouse (655) and an anti-abortifacient action in the rat (656). The abortion-inhibiting action of progestins has been the subject of many studies [81, 88 (Ch. 2), 657, 658]. Most remarkable perhaps is the action of progestin-estrogen administration in maintaining pregnancy in rats on a protein-free diet. This exogenous support, or support by endogenous ovarian hormone stimulated by a combination of FSH, LH, and LTH, overcomes what would otherwise be complete sterility (659). It is notable in this regard that non-ovulating, undernourished rats form corpora lutea promptly on rehabilitation (660). Hormone responses in such animals and similarly sterile, undernourished pigs (661) would be much worth examining.

REFERENCES

495. Fawcett, D. W., Wislocki, G. B., and Waldo, C. M. 1947. *Am. J. Anat.* **81**, 413.
496. Runner, M. N. 1947. *Anat. Record* **18**, 1.
497. Ahlgren, M., and Bengtsson, L. P. 1962. *J. Reprod. Fertility* **3**, 89.
498. Nicholas, S. J. 1942. *J. Exptl. Zool.* **90**, 41.
499. Kirby, D. R. S. 1960. *Nature* **194**, 785.
500. Kirby, D. R. S., 1963. *J. Reprod. Fertility* **5**, 1.
501. Tarkowski, A. K. 1962. *J. Embryol. Exptl. Morphol.* **10**, 476.
502. Averill, R. W. L., Adams, C. E., and Rowson, L. E. A. 1955. *Nature* **179**, 238.
503. Hafez, E. S. E., and Sugie, T. 1963. *J. Animal Sci.* **22**, 30.
504. Lutwak-Mann, C., Hay, M. F., and Adams, C. E. 1962. *J. Endocrinol.* **24**, 185.
505. Kirby, D. R. S. 1962. *J. Embryol. Exptl. Morphol.* **10**, 496.
506. Chang, M. C. 1950. *J. Exptl. Zool.* **114**, 197.
507. Dickmann, Z., and Noyes, R. W. 1960. *J. Reprod. Fertility* **1**, 197.
508. Enders, A. C., ed. 1963. "Delayed Implantation." Univ. of Chicago Press, Chicago, Illinois.
509. Enzmann, E. V., Saphir, N. R., and Pincus, G. 1932. *Anat. Record* **54**, 275.
510. Whitten, W. K. 1958. *J. Endocrinol.* **16**, 435.
511. Boving, B. G. 1963. *In* "Mechanisms Concerned with Conception" (C. G. Hartman, ed.), p. 321. Macmillan, New York.
512. Ramsey, E. M. 1960. *In* "Les Fonctions de Nidation Uterine et Leurs Troubles," p. 153. Masson et Cie, Paris.
513. Noyes, R. W., Adams, C. E., and Walton, A. 1959. *J. Endocrinol.* **18**, 108.
514. Noyes, R. W., Dickmann, Z., Doyle, L. L., and Gates, A. H. 1963. *In* "Delayed Implantation" (A. C. Enders, ed.), p. 197. Univ. of Chicago Press, Chicago, Illinois.
515. Cochrane, R. L., and Meyer, R. K. 1957. *Proc. Soc. Exptl. Biol. Med.* **96**, 155.
516. Canívenc, R., and Lafarque, M. 1957. *Compt. Rend. Acad. Sci.* **254**, 1752.

517. Mayer, G. 1959. *In* "Implantation of Ova" (P. Eckstein, ed.), p. 76. Cambridge Univ. Press, London and New York.

518. Psychoyos, A., and Alloiteau, J. J. 1962. *Compt. Rend. Soc. Biol.* **156,** 46.

519. Zeilmaker, G. H. 1963. *Acta Endocrinol.* **44,** 355.

520. Psychoyos, A. 1963. *J. Endocrinol.* **27,** 337.

521. Mayer, G. 1963. *In* "Delayed Implantation" (A. C. Enders, ed.), p. 213. Univ. of Chicago Press, Chicago, Illinois.

522. Nutting, E. F., and Meyer, R. K. 1964. *Endocrinology* **74,** 573.

523. Nutting, E. F., and Meyer, R. K. 1964. *J. Endocrinol.* **29,** 235.

524. Buchanan, G. D., Enders, A. C., and Talmage, R. V. 1956. *J. Endocrinol.* **14,** 121.

525. Enders, A. C. 1961. *Am. Zool.* **1,** 447.

526. Meyer, R. K., and Cochrane, R. L. 1962. *J. Endocrinol.* **24,** 77.

527. Orsini, M. W., and Meyer, R. K. 1962. *Proc. Soc. Exptl. Biol. Med.* **110,** 713.

528. Czyba, J. C. 1963. *Compt. Rend. Acad. Sci.* **256,** 2242.

529. Shelesnyak, M. C. 1963. *J. Reprod. Fertility* **5,** 295.

530. Shelesnyak, M. C. 1964. *In* "Techniques in Endocrine Research," p. 231. Academic Press, New York.

531. Blandau, R. J. 1949. *Anat. Record* **104,** 331.

532. Böving, B. G. 1959. *Ann. N. Y. Acad. Sci.* **75,** 700.

533. Spaziani, E., and Szego, C. M. 1958. *Endocrinology* **63,** 669.

534. Shelesnyak, M. C., Kraicer, P. F., and Zeilmaker, G. H. 1963. *Acta Endocrinol.* **42,** 225.

535. Marcus, G. J., Kraicer, P. F., and Shelesnyak, M. C. 1963. *J. Reprod. Fertility* **5,** 409.

536. Shelesnyak, M. C. 1957. *Recent Progr. Hormone Res.* **13,** 269.

537. Kraicer, P. F., Marcus, G. J., and Shelesnyak, M. C. 1963. *J. Reprod. Fertility* **5,** 417.

538. Shelesnyak, M. C., and Tic, L. 1963. *Acta Endocrinol.* **43,** 462.

539. Orsini, M. W. 1963. *J. Reprod. Fertility* **5,** 323.

540. Chambon, Y. 1961. *Compt. Rend. Soc. Biol.* **155,** 1351.

541. Finn, C. A., and Keen, P. M. 1962. *Nature* **194,** 602.

542. Banik, U. K., and Ketchel, M. M. 1964. *J. Reprod. Fertility* **7,** 259.

543. Finn, C. A., and Emmens, C. W. 1961. *J. Reprod. Fertility* **2,** 528.

544. Hisaw, F. L., and Velardo, J. T. 1951. *Endocrinology* **49,** 530.

545. Lerner, L. J., Holthaus, F. J., Jr., and Thompson, C. R. 1958. *Endocrinology* **59,** 306.

546. Emmens, C. W. 1963. *J. Reprod. Fertility* **5,** 292.

547. Banik, U. K., Kobayashi, Y., and Ketchel, M. M. 1963. *J. Reprod. Fertility* **6,** 179.

548. Finn, C. A., and Keen, P. M. 1962. *J. Endocrinol.* **24,** 381.

549. Glenister, T. W. 1962. *J. Obstet. Gynaecol.* **69,** 809.

550. Kar, A. B., and Sen, D. P. 1962. *Gerontologia* **6,** 144.

551. Fernandez-Cano, L. 1959. *In* "Endocrinology of Reproduction" (C. W. Lloyd, ed.), p. 97. Academic Press, New York.

552. Giuliani, G., Martini, L., Pecile, A., and Fochi, M. 1961. *Acta Endocrinol.* 38, 1.

553. Courrier, R., and Collonge, A. 1951. *J. Am. Med. Assoc.* 146, 493.

554. Gabka, J., and Hassiotis, J. 1962. *J. Arztl. Forsch.* 16, 541.

555. Robson, J. M., and Sharaf, A. A. 1952. *J. Physiol. (London)* 116, 236.

556. Wexler, B. C. 1964. *Endocrinology* 74, 65.

557. Lindsay, D., Poulson, E., and Robson, J. M. 1961. *J. Endocrinol.* 23, 209.

558. Poulson, E., and Robson, J. M. 1963. *Brit. J. Pharmacol.* 21, 150.

559. Lutwak-Mann, C. 1959. *In* "Implantation of Ova" (P. Eckstein, ed.), p. 35. Cambridge Univ. Press, London and New York.

560. Pincus, G., and Bialy, G. 1963. *Recent Progr. Hormone Res.* 19, 201.

561. Prahlad, K. V. 1962. *Acta Endocrinol.* 34, 407.

562. Leone, E., Libonati, M., and Lutwak-Mann, C. 1963. *J. Endocrinol.* 25, 551.

563. Rosa, C. G., and Velardo, J. T. 1959. *Ann. N. Y. Acad. Sci.* 75, 491.

564. Fishman, W. H., and Fishman, L. W. 1944. *J. Biol. Chem.* 152, 487.

565. Albers, H. J., and Castro, M. E. 1961. *Fertility Sterility* 12, 142.

566. Hafez, E. S. E. 1964. *Acta Endocrinol.* 46, 217.

567. Gregoire, A. T., Eongsakü, D., and Rakoff, A. E. 1962. *Fertility Sterility* 13, 432.

568. Vishwakarma, P. 1962. *Fertility Sterility* 13, 481.

569. Böving, B. G. 1959. *In* "Endocrinology of Reproduction" (C. W. Lloyd, ed.), p. 205. Academic Press, New York.

570. Madjerek, Z., and van de Vies, J. 1961. *Acta Endocrinol.* 38, 315.

571. Ogawa, Y., and Pincus, G. 1962. *Endocrinology* 70, 359.

572. Lutwak-Mann, C. 1962. *Nature* 193, 653.

573. Eckstein, P., Shelesnyak, M. C., and Amoroso, E. C. 1959. *In* "Implantation of Ova" (P. Eckstein, ed.), p. 3. Cambridge Univ. Press, London and New York.

574. Hammond, J. 1952. *In* "Physiology of Reproduction" (A. S. Parkes, ed.), p. 648. Longmans Green, London.

575. Gordon, I. 1958. *J. Agr. Sci.* 50, 123.

576. McLaren, A., and Michie, D. 1959. *J. Exptl. Biol.* 36, 281.

577. Wilson, E. D., and Edwards, R. G. 1963. *J. Reprod. Fertility* 5, 179.

578. Hayward, J. N., Hilliard, J., and Sawyer, C. H. 1963. *Proc. Soc. Exptl. Biol. Med.* 113, 256.

579. Short, R. V., McDonald, M. F., and Rowson, L. E. A. 1963. *J. Endocrinol.* 26, 155.

580. Hafez, E. S. E., ed. 1962. *In* "Reproduction in Farm Animals," p. 111. Lea & Febiger, Philadelphia.

581. Wislocki, G. B., and Snyder, F. F. 1933. *Bull. Johns Hopkins Hosp.* 35, 246.

582. Greenwald, G. S. 1961. *Endocrinology* 69, 1068.

583. Greenwald, G. S. 1959. *Fertility Sterility* 10, 155.
584. Deansley, R. 1961. *Proc. Intern. Congr. Animal Reprod.* 2, 371.
585. Deansley, R. 1963. *J. Reprod. Fertility* 5, 49.
586. Edgren, R. A., Petersen, D., Johnson, M. A., and Shipley, G. C. 1961. *Fertility Sterility* 12, 172.
587. Edgren, R. A., and Shipley, G. C. 1961. *Fertility Sterility* 12, 179.
588. Martin, L. 1963. *J. Endocrinol.* 26, 31.
589. Stone, G. M., and Emmens, C. W. 1964. *J. Endocrinol.* 29, 147.
590. Emmens, C. W. 1962. *J. Reprod. Fertility* 3, 246.
591. Martin, L., Cox, R. I., and Emmens, C. W. 1963. *J. Reprod. Fertility* 5, 239.
592. Stone, G. M., and Emmens, C. W. 1964. *J. Endocrinol.* 29, 137.
593. Emmens, C. W., Cox, R. I., and Martin, L. 1964. *Acta Endocrinol. Suppl.* 90, 61.
594. Lerner, L. J., Turkheimer, A. R., and Borman, A. 1963. *Proc. Soc. Exptl. Biol. Med.* 114, 115.
595. Leathem, J. H., and Adams, W. C. 1961. *Federation Proc.* 20, 198.
596. Lednicer, D., Babcock, J. C., Lyster, S. C., Stucki, J. C., and Duncan, G. W. 1961. *Chem. Ind.* (*London*) p. 2098.
597. Duncan, G. W., and Lyster, S. C. 1962. *Federation Proc.* 21, 437.
598. Lednicer, D., Babcock, J. C. Lyster, S. C., and Duncan, G. W. 1963. *Chem. & Ind.* (*London*) p. 408.
599. Duncan, G. W., Lyster, S. C., Clark, J. J., and Lednicer, D. 1963. *Proc. Soc. Exptl. Biol. Med.* 112, 439.
600. Nelson, W. O., Davidson, O. W., and Wada, K. 1963. *In* "Delayed Implantation" (A. C. Enders, ed.), p. 183. Univ. of Chicago Press, Chicago, Illinois.
601. Sanyal, S. N. 1959. *J. Med. Intern. Med. Abstr.* 23, 15.
602. Prahlad, K. V., and Kar, A. B. 1963. *Fertility Sterility* 14, 372.
603. Psychoyos, A. 1963. *Compt. Rend. Acad. Sci.* 257, 1367.
604. Nutting, E. F., and Meyer, R. K. 1962. *Proc. Soc. Exptl. Biol. Med.* 111, 372.
605. Cochrane, R. L., and Shackleford, R. M. 1962. *J. Endocrinol.* 25, 101.
606. Davis, B. K. 1963. *Nature* 157, 308.
607. Saunders, F. J., and Elton, R. L. 1959. *In* "Endocrinology of Reproduction" (C. W. Lloyd, ed.), p. 227. Academic Press, New York.
608. Edgren, R. A., and Smith, H. 1962. *1st Intern. Congr. Hormonal Steroids, Milan* p. 68.
609. Clauberg, C. 1930. *Zentr. Gynaekol.* 54, 2757.
610. Yamashita, K., and Kuronji, K. 1961. *Proc. Soc. Exptl. Biol. Med.* 107, 444.
611. Yamashita, K., and Kuronji, K. I. 1961. *Nature* 190, 1013.
612. Banik, U. K., and Pincus, G. 1962. *Proc. Soc. Exptl. Biol. Med.* 111, 595.
613. Pincus, G., Banik, U., and Jacques, J. 1964. *Steroids* 4, 657.

614. Saunders, F. J., and Rorig, K. 1964. *Fertility Sterility* 15, 202.
615. Barnes, L. E., and Meyer, R. K. 1962. *Fertility Sterility* 13, 472.
616. Carlsen, R. A., Zeilmaker, G. H., and Shelesnyak, M. C. 1961. *J. Reprod. Fertility* 2, 369.
617. Shelesnyak, M. C., and Barnes, A. 1963. *Acta Endocrinol.* 43, 469.
618. Robson, J. M. 1959. *In* "Implantation of Ova" (P. Eckstein, ed.), p. 54. Cambridge Univ. Press, London and New York.
619. Jackson, D., and Robson, J. M. 1957. *J. Endocrinol.* 14, 348.
620. Lutwak-Mann, C., and Hay, M. F. 1962. *Brit. Med. J.* I, p. 944.
621. Popp, R. A. 1958. *J. Exptl. Zool.* 138, 1.
622. Chamberlain, J. 1963. *Anat. Record* 145, 312.
623. Joshi, M. S., Patwardhan, V. V., and Panse, T. B. 1963. *J. Reprod. Fertility* 5, 288.
624. Hafez, E. S. E., and Pincus, G. 1956. *Fertility Sterility* 7, 422.
625. Meyer, R. K., and Cochrane, R. L. 1962. *J. Reprod. Fertility* 4, 67.
626. Doyle, L. L., and Margolis, A. J. 1963. *Science* 139, 833.
627. Zipper, J. A., Delgado, R., and Guiloff, E. 1964. Unpublished data.
628. Carleton, H., and Phelps, H. 1933. *J. Obstet. Gynaecol. Brit. Empire* 40, 81.
629. Chatterjee, S. N., and Luktake, S. N. 1961. *J. Reprod. Fertility* 2, 196.
630. Parkes, A. S. 1963. *In* "Perspectives in Biology" (Cori, Foglia, Leloir, and Ochoa, eds.), p. 33. Elsevier, London.
631. Bruce, H. M. 1962. *J. Reprod. Fertility* 4, 313.
632. Parkes, A. S., and Bruce, H. M. 1962. *J. Reprod. Fertility* 4, 303.
633. Marsden, H. M., and Bronson, F. H. 1964. *Science* 144, 1469.
634. Zonhar, R. L., and de Groot, J. 1963. *Anat. Record* 145, 358.
635. Flament-Durand, J., and Desclin, L. 1964. *Endocrinology* 75, 22.
636. Armstrong, D. T., and Hansel, W. 1959. *J. Dairy Sci.* 42, 533.
637. Simmon, K. R., and Hansel, W. 1964. *J. Animal Sci.* 23, 136.
638. Brinkley, H. J., Norton, H. W., and Nalbandov, A. V. 1964. *Endocrinology* 74, 9.
639. Nishikawa, Y., and Horie, T. 1963. *Proc. Japan Acad.* 39, 764.
640. Greenwald, G. S. 1964. *Am. Zool.* 4, 281.
641. Harper, M. J. K. 1964. *J. Reprod. Fertility* 7, 211.
642. Saunders, F. J. 1964. *Acta Endocrinol.* 46, 157.
643. Davis, B. K. 1963. *J. Endocrinol.* 27, 99.
644. Barnes, L. E., and Meyer, R. K. 1964. *J. Reprod. Fertility* 7, 139.
645. Hayashida, T., and Young, W. P. 1963. *Anat. Record* 145, 323.
646. Young, W. P., Nasser, R., and Hayashida, T. 1963. *Anat. Record* 145, 357.
647. Blaha, G. C. 1963. *Anat. Record* 145, 208.
648. Thiersch, J. B. 1962. *J. Reprod. Fertility* 4, 291.
649. Thiersch, J. B. 1962. *J. Reprod. Fertility* 4, 297.
650. Lindsay, D., Paulson, E., and Robson, J. M. 1963. *J. Endocrinol.* 26, 85.
651. Robson, J. M., and Sullivan, F. M. 1963. *J. Endocrinol.* 25, 553.

652. Kameswaran, L., Pennefeather, J. N., and West, G. P. 1962. *J. Physiol.* (*London*) **164**, 138.
653. Marois, M. 1960. *Compt. Rend. Soc. Biol.* **154**, 1361.
654. Rahlmann, D. F., and Cupps, P. T. 1962. *J. Dairy Sci.* **45**, 1003.
655. Hoshino, K. 1963. *Anat. Record* **145**, 327.
656. Dessarzin, D., and Stamm, O. 1962. *Gynaecologia* **154**, 272.
657. Csapo, A. 1956. *Recent Progr. Hormone Res.* **12**, 405.
658. Fuchs, F., and Koch, F. 1963. *Acta Endocrinol.* **42**, 403.
659. Kinzey, W. G., and Skrebnik, H. H. 1963. *Anat. Record* **145**, 249.
660. Widdowson, E. M., Mavor, W. O., and McCance, R. A. 1964. *J. Endocrinol.* **29**, 119.
661. Dickerson, J. W. T., Gresham, G. A., and McCance, R. A. 1964. *J. Endocrinol.* **29**, 111.

CHAPTER 8

Some Biological Activities of Compounds Affecting Fertility

Many of the substances or preparations described in the preceding chapters have rather limited effects in animals, e.g., specific antibodies, erucic acid, antifertilizin. Others have primary physiological or pharmacological effects on tissues and processes not concerned with reproduction, e.g., tranquilizers, some of the antimetabolites. Then there are compounds with demonstrated antifertility effects, but with either unknown biological potencies or rather mysterious ones. As an example of the former we cite the guanylhydrazones (*662*) which are active sterilizing agents in both male and female rats, *perhaps* as antifolic agents, but lacking the toxicity of the usual antifolics (e.g., aminopterin). The presently mysterious one is N-acetylneuraminic acid which inhibits PMS-HCG-induced superovulation in mice (*663*), and which has a toxicity at high dose suggestive of antimetabolite action. Most of the substances discussed, however, have various physiological properties affecting particularly endocrine functions. Those most studied have been the steroids. Since they are such powerful agents affecting reproduction, it is natural that their involvement in a variety of related and unrelated processes be examined. For antifertility agents, such involvements may afford information relative to significant side effects.

To detail all of the biological activities of the steroids would require an effort quite beyond the scope of this book. Such an effort has indeed been made by Applezweig (*664*) who has coded some 1500 steroids and classified them into 21 categories of biological activity (Table 25). The role of fertility-affecting steroids in these various types of activity is often unexpected. Since many of them have wide repercussive effects, i.e., as the result of actions on other endocrine organs, effects on the thresholds of tissue activity, etc., etc., an often bewildering set of functions is attributed

TABLE 25

SOME BIOLOGICAL ACTIVITIES OF STEROIDS[a]

Anabolic	Anti-androgen
Androgen	Antibacteria
Active on circulatory system	Anticancer
Corticoid	Anticorticoid
Active on central nervous system	Antimineralocorticoid (diuretic)
Estrogen	Anti-estrogen
Lipodiatic	Antifungus
Mineralocorticoid	Antigonadotropin
Progestogen	Anti-osteoporotic
Miscellaneous	Antiprogestogen
	Antivirus

[a] From Applezweig (*664*).

to them. Thus estrogen administration has been followed in one species or another by measurable effects on either the growth or on aspects of the metabolism of practically every tissue of the mammalian body (cf. *665*). Nonetheless, certain functions of these active compounds are worthy of note where they involve effects of possible pertinence to their roles in reproductive processes.

Some Activities of Estrogens

Among the most studied of the natural estrogens—estradiol, estrone, and estriol—certain differences, both qualitative and quantitative, have been repeatedly emphasized in animal experiments. Since estrone and estradiol are rather freely intraconvertible *in vivo*, their biological activities tend generally to be quite similar with the former usually exhibiting lesser potency. In mice estradiol is more tightly bound to uterine tissue than estrone (*666*) and this appears to be true also for several tissues in the guinea pig

(*667*). This may account for its higher activity. Estriol, which is a product of estrone metabolism (*668, 669*), generally shows rather large quantitative differences from its precursor and may be inactive in target tissues in which estrone is quite active (*670*). In stimulating uterine weight increase in immature female rats, estriol has high activity at low dose but fails to yield the maximal growth stimulation afforded by estrone and estradiol (*671*). As an inhibitor of gonadotropin secretion in parabiotic rats, estriol has $\frac{1}{40}$ to $\frac{1}{50}$ the activity of estradiol (*672*). According to Genet *et al.* (*673*) it acts just like estrone in its inhibition of FSH at low dose and stimulation of LH at high dose, but its presumed immediate metabolic precursor, 16-hydroxyestrone, although similarly uterotrophic, has no effect on the release or production of pituitary gonadotropins. Velardo (*674*) has shown that estriol (and its isomer 16-epiestriol) acts as a pacemaker on simultaneous injection with the other natural estrogens. This competitive inhibition by estriol is abolished when it is administered at its 3-cyclopentyl ether to mice along with estrone (*675*); furthermore its dose: response curve rises steeply to maximal levels instead of plateauing off at mid-level.

Other distinctions among the natural estrogens as effector agents may be gleaned from the reviews of Velardo (*674*) and Pincus (*676*). Similarly, the many synthetic estrogens will mimic and yet differ in one respect or another from the natural estrogens. Huggins and Jensen (*677*) have introduced the term "impeded estrogens" to describe the oxygenated estrogens that modify estrone effects on the uterus. We have noted that such compounds may differentially affect ovum development and/or uterine response (*vide supra*). Velardo (*674, 678*) has advanced the concept that the regulatory activity of the estrogens, particularly upon the uterus, is normally modified by other hormones and that "the metabolic alterations of the uterus are due to all of the hormones and their metabolites in concert." He cites not only estrogen interactions affecting uterine growth, but also progesterone antagonism and synergism, inhibitions of estradiol action by testosterone and various corticoids. Similar reactions with thyroid hormone have been reviewed by Leathem (*679*). Recently the pineal gland has been involved as the source of a specific inhibitor of estrogen action on uterus and vagina (*680, 681*). The effects of pinealectomy have, however, been ascribed at least in part to a pineal-pituitary axis (*682*). The upset of this complex equilibrium by altering any one of the factors contributed to it would then appear to be the basis of much, if not all,

TABLE 26

EFFECT OF STEROIDS ON RAT UTERINE LDH-DPNH OXIDASE ACTIVITY[a]

| | Relative enzyme activities | | | |
| | Effect of steroid alone | | Effect of steroid given with estradiol | |
Steroid	LDH	DPNH oxidase	LDH	DPNH oxidase
(1) Estradiol-17β	+++	++++	−	—
(2) Estrone	++	+++	− −	Additive effect
(3) Estriol	++++	++	?	Estriol inhib. estradiol − − − −
(4) Progesterone	+++++	− −	Estradiol inhib. prog. − − −	Prog. inhib. estradiol − − − −
(5) DCA	++++	+++	Estradiol inhib. DCA − − − −	DCA inhib. estradiol − − −
(6) Testosterone	++	++	Estradiol inhib. test. − − − −	Test. inhib. estradiol − −
(7) Cortisone acetate	±	+	Estradiol inhib. cort. − −	No effect

[a] From Bever (*683*).

of the sterilizing actions of agents acting on the uterus. What then is the basic uterine biochemistry to which these hormonal factors contribute their influences?

As an example of the effects on uterine tissue activity we present in Table 26 Bever's (*683*) summary of the effects upon rat uterine lactic dehydrogenase (LDH) and reduced diphosphopyridine nucleotide (DPNH) oxidase of various hormonal steroids and their interactions with estradiol. The most potent stimulator of

DPNH oxidase activity is estradiol, whereas progesterone is most active in stimulating LDH activity. The various interactions of these steroids upon these enzymes do not per se explain interactions on growth and various other metabolic events. Indeed, numerous enzyme systems in the uterus are steroid labile (684, 685). In fact, differential effects of estrogens on various enzyme systems may occur in the vagina and uterus or even in different parts of the uterus. Thus in ovariectomized rats, estradiol administration increases vaginal concentrations of β-glucuronidase, esterase, and alkaline phosphatase within 2 hours, but with no notable change in acid phosphatase. The acid phosphatase increases rapidly in the uterus as does esterase and alkaline phosphatase. β-Glucuronidase concentration in the uterine endometrium increases, but decreases in the epithelium (686). We have already indicated (p. 119) that many other uterine enzyme systems are affected by hormonal steroids. Generally the effects of estrogen are opposed by progesterone, e.g., the phosphorylase increase in the inner circular layer of the rat uterus (687), the increased β-glucuronidase activity in mouse uteri (688), or by synthetic gestagens (689). The 5-nucleotidase activity in mouse uteri has been reported as unresponsive to estrogens, but significantly increased in pseudopregnancy and after progesterone administration (690). Since practically all metabolic events occurring in the organs of the reproductive tract must be enzyme-mediated, it is natural to ascribe to hormonal effects on enzyme systems the significant basis of their action. It is difficult, however, to decide what are the primary events in hormone action and what are the secondary, tertiary, etc., outcomes of their initial action.

The obvious initial event in the action of any hormone is its means of entry and localization in the target tissue. In the case of the estrogens this has been studied by examining the uptake of radioactive estrogen, and a high concentration in target tissues appears to be due primarily to prolonged retention (691, 692). Gestagens and the anti-estrogen MER-25 (but not DMS) prevent the uptake of radioactive estradiol into the rodent uterus and vagina (692, 693). Only MER-25 was active in such inhibition on vaginal inunction; interestingly the gestagen 17α-ethyl-19-nortestosterone acted locally to hasten the departure of accumulated vaginal estrogen (694) as did DMS (695). Whether the target tissue binding protein is part of the "active" complex or merely a transfer agent remains to be determined.

The problem of the mechanism of action of the steroid hormones has been extensively discussed in numerous publications (*684, 685, 696–698*). Explanations of their actions vary for each type of steroid, but five general controlling effects have been postulated at one time or another: (a) alteration of the rate of synthesis of new enzyme, (b) conversion of "inactive" enzyme to active enzyme, (c) action as a cofactor in an enzyme system, (d) competition with essential cofactor(s), and (e) alteration of cellular or subcellular particle permeability.

A general theory attempting to account for all hormone action originally expressed by Karlson (*699*) and Zalokar (*700*) is that the regulation of genetic programming by hormones is the immediate cause of enzyme formation and consequent alterations in cellular metabolism. This concept has recently been reviewed critically by Hechter and Halkerston (*701*), and some of its possible modes of operation are presented diagrammatically in Fig. 14. Most frequently studied in this connection has been the action of estrogen upon the uterus, particularly in ovariectomized animals. Following estrogen administration, uterine increases in RNA polymerase (*702*), in messenger RNA (*703*), and in transfer RNA (*704*) have been claimed, and the blocking of estrogen-stimulated RNA synthesis in the uterus by puromycin (*705*) and actinomycin D (*706*) has been noted. These findings may indeed be interpreted as a direct action of estrogen, but the possibility that estrogen plus a receptor produce a "key" protein which in turn activates the RNA mechanisms has been considered more likely (*701, 707*). Pointing out that water imbibition and uterine growth are two major "primary" effects of estrogen on the rodent uterus which may be independently influenced, i.e., the former is labile to administered corticosteroid (*708*); whereas RNA, protein, and phospholipid synthesis are not (*709*), Hechter and Halkerston suggest caution in considering that there is a single hormone-generated event responsible for all of the estrogen-induced effects. Indeed a possibility of specific reactions in each of the several types of uterine tissue has not been explored.

Such specific mechanisms have been described in various in-

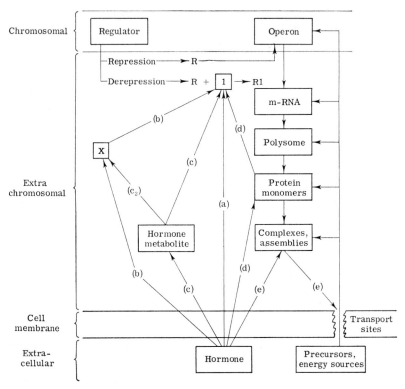

FIG. 14. Diagrammatic representation of possible sites of hormone participation in gene activity and protein synthesis. In the chromosomes the operon
(usually considered to be DNA) is responsible for the RNA polymerase producing messenger RNA (m-RNA) which acts upon polysomes responsible for
protein monomer formation and eventual protein complexes or macromolecular
assemblies. The chromosomal regulator is responsible for the production of
repressor substance (R) which must combine with inducer (I) to allow the
operon to express itself in terms of m-RNA. Hormones may stimulate protein
synthesis by acting directly as inducers (route a) and/or they may act as the
gene locus, inhibiting regulator activity. A precursor, or binding site, X, for I
may be hormone-controlled (route b), or a hormone metabolite may be the
key substance to the evocation of X (route C_2) or action on I (route c).
Hormone might affect the transcription of the messenger RNA at the poly-
ribosomal site producing an abnormal protein which feeds back to induce
derepression (route d). Route e suggests the possibility of hormone alteration
of the complexes and macromolecular assemblies causing secondary changes
influencing precursor availability and hence gene expressivity (*701*).

stances, e.g., new synthesis of enzyme under influence of estrogen [*560* (Ch. 7), *685*] or androgen (*710, 711*), the activation of placental transhydrogenase by estrogen (*712*). The "primary event" in estrogen action has been denominated as an increased tissue concentration of the biogenic amines histamine [*533* (Ch. 7)], serotonin (*713*), adrenaline (*714*), which may be released from intrauterine binding by reserpine (*715*), or of "active" transhydrogenase (*712*). The increased active amine has been attributed in the guinea pig to mast cell degranulation on acute estrogen administration (*716*), which may be inhibited by alloxan administration (*717*). As in the case of deciduomagenic action, histamine has been challenged as the evoker of water imbibition (or glycogen increases), since its intraluminal instillation does not lead to these events (*718*). Thus the antifertility effects of such diverse agents as monoamine oxidase inhibitors, chelating agents, anti-estrogens, certain enzyme poisons, would all seem to relate to the basic processes initiated by the sex hormones.

Anti-estrogens

In view of the foregoing, it is not surprising that the search for anti-estrogens as potential antifertility agents is a most active one. Dorfman and Kincl (*719*) have recently reported on a large series of synthetic steroids as inhibitors of the estrone-stimulated uterine hypertrophy in immature mice. Out of a large number tested, activity at doses 5 to 200 times the standard estrogen dose was shown by 23 compounds listed in Table 27. Among the progestational steroids tested, no meaningful correlation could be detected between progestational potency in the Clauberg assay and anti-estrogenic activity, e.g., compound XXI in oral assay is the most potent progestin having 35 times the potency of the standard norethisterone (III) but it is only one third as active as norethisterone as an anti-estrogen. Apparently minor molecular modifications often abolished detectable anti-estrogenic activity, e.g., the substitution of fluorine for chlorine at carbon 6 in compound XXI or the substitution of a 6β Cl for the 6α Cl of compound XXII. Other steroidal anti-estrogens have been described by Dorfman [*199* (Ch. 3), *720*] and interesting new types by Loken *et al.* (*721*), Hecker and

TABLE 27
HIGHLY ACTIVE ANTI-ESTROGENS

Compound no.	Steroid	Minimum dose to produce inhibition, μg (maximum inhibition %)	
		Subcutaneous injection	Gavage
I	2α,17α-Dimethyl-17β-hydroxy-5α-androstan-3-one	2(30)[a]	
II	17α-Ethyl-19-nortestosterone	8(54)[a]	40(43)[b]
III	17α-Ethynyl-19-nortestosterone	16(56)[a]	32(40)[b]
IV	17α-Methyl-19-nortestosterone	32(46)[a]	40(44)[b]
V	17α-Methyltestosterone	32(35)[a]	
VI	2α-Methyl-17β-hydroxy-5α-androstan-3-one	50(47)[a]	
VII	17α-Methyl-17β-hydroxy-5α-19-norandrostan-3-one	50(38)[a]	
VIII	6α,16α-Dimethylprogesterone	5(60)	
IX	6α-Fluoro-16α-methylprogesterone	10(61)	50(63)
X	6α-Fluoroprogesterone	10(34)	
XI	6β,16α-Dimethylprogesterone	20(53)	10(55)
XII	6β,16α-Dimethyl-5α-hydroxy-pregnane-3,20-dione	30(18)	
XIII	6β-Fluoro-16α-methylprogesterone	50(44)	50(32)
XIV	4-Chloro-19-norprogesterone	50(47)	
XV	17α-Acetoxy-19-norprogesterone		50(21)
XVI	17α-Acetoxyprogesterone	25(39)	
XVII	6α-Fluoro-17α-acetoxyprogesterone	50(50)	
XVIII	6-Chloro-16α-methyl-Δ⁶-dehydro-17α-acetoxyprogesterone	50(52)	
XIX	6α,16α-Dimethyl-17α-acetoxyprogesterone	50(52)	
XX	6-Chloro-Δ¹·⁶-bisdehydro-17α-acetoxyprogesterone	50(49)	
XXI	6-Chloro-Δ⁶-dehydro-17α-acetoxyprogesterone	50(40)	
XXII	6α-Chloro-17α-acetoxyprogesterone	80(56)	80(28)
XXIII	2-Cyano-5α-androst-2-en-17β-ol	10(45)	

[a] Data of Dorfman and Kincl (719).
[b] Data of Dorfman (720).

Farthofer (722), and Edgren et al. (723). A simple test for anti-estrogenic activity has recently been proposed by Lee and Williams (724). Estrone (40 μg per liter) in the drinking water of mice causes a constant vaginal cornification which is inhibited by a single injection of gestagen.

Of the nonsteroidal anti-estrogens we have already discussed stilbestrol derivatives investigated principally by Emmens and his colleagues. A rather peculiar anti-estrogenic effect of β-glycyrrhetinic acid in rats has been described by Kraus (725), who finds it inhibits the action of exogenous but not of endogenous estrogen even when the latter is stimulated by exogenous gonadotropin. A similar inhibition by N,N'-diphenyl-p-phenylenediamine (DPPD) of the action of exogenous but not endogenous estrogen has been reported (726). DPPD actually lengthens pregnancy when administered per os or subcutaneously in a single dose to gravid rats (727). Adler (728) finds an active anti-estrogen in alfalfa leaf extracts which, he believes, accounts for the low incidence of mammary carcinoma in cows and sheep. It may be that a similar substance causing vaginal estrus but often inhibiting behavioral estrus is responsible for the fertilized egg degeneration seen in animals fed a diet rich in leguminous forage (729). An aqueous extract of pine needles contains a quite potent anti-estrogen (730). The diabetes due to alloxan administration to rats but not that caused by pancreatectomy markedly diminishes uterine responsivity to estrogen. This suggested the evocation of an endogenous anti-estrogen. Since adrenalectomy corrects the depression of activity an adrenocortical secretion product is suggested (731). ACTH injected into mice has a marked inhibitory effect on ovarian growth, prevents ovulation and estrus. Since this effect is seen in adrenalectomized mice maintained on corticosteroid, a direct action on the ovaries is suggested.

Indeed, estrogen-corticosteroid antagonism has long been known and both mineralocorticoids and glucocorticoids have been demonstrably potent anti-estrogens (674, 678). This antagonism may be demonstrated on uterine hydration with cortisol injection within 2 hours of estrogen administration (733). Cortisone administration will reduce the number and extent of hepatic lesions induced by high doses of estrogen. In turn, the estrogen prevents cortisone-induced sclerosis of the reticular zone of the adrenal cortex (734). Conservation of adrenal resources by endogenous ovarian hormone is indicated by the finding that in ovariectomized rats examined up to 8 months following castration, adrenal corticosterone was significantly less in concentration and in total quantity per gland although no significant adrenal weight loss took place (735). Replacement therapy in ovariectomized rats increases plasma and adrenal corticosterone and also pituitary ACTH (736).

Estrogens and Androgens

The sterilizing effect of estrogen injected into newborn rats (737) may be due to a stimulation of the pituitary adrenal axis since it is marked by pituitary hypertrophy with growth inhibition and thymus atrophy, the latter a typical effect of adrenocortical hyperactivity. The accompanying retardation of vaginal opening, ovarian atrophy, and lack of female sex behavior have been known for some time (738, 739), and replacement therapy has not led to normal mating behavior (740). This has led to the concept of feminization and of action on a mating-behavior center in the brain (741). The degree of effect is dose proportional with either estrone (742) or estradiol benzoate administration (743). A hormone-conditioned type of gonad-controlling pattern is suggested by data from male rats castrated shortly after birth. Such animals appear to retain the female pattern of pituitary hormone release since ovaries transplanted to them in adulthood exhibit cyclic ovulation and corpus luteum formation (739, 744, 745), and concomitant vaginal implants show the usual 4-day cycle (746). In male rats castrated at 2 days of age and receiving on day 5 either testosterone propionate or estradiol benzoate injection, such ovarian transplants exhibit no cyclicity and fail to form corpora lutea (745). Estradiol benzoate in single injection (of 0.12 mg) administered to 5-day-old male rats is clearly sterilizing, causing inhibition of spermatogenesis and testis and accessory gland atrophy; this effect on sexual organ development does not occur if the estrogen is administered 5 or 15 days later (746).

This notion of an undifferentiated neural mechanism in 1- to 5-day-old rats has been reinforced by the sterilizing action of androgen administered to newborn female rats which in adulthood exhibit constant vaginal estrus (739), lack of female mating behavior, and a male pattern if ovariectomy and testosterone proprionate administration is practiced (747, 748). The lack of ovulation in these rats appears to be due to a reduction of pituitary LH. The restoration of ovulation has been accomplished by priming with progesterone which acts to increase pituitary LH and then electrically stimulating the median eminence so as to induce adequate LH release (*743, 749*). Pregnant mare's serum (PMS) alone fails to ovulate these androgen-sterilized females, but PMS plus HCG causes the usual superovulation (*750*) and FSH plus HCG is similarly effective (*751*), again suggesting endogenous LH lack. A hypothalamic locus is suggested by lesions in the mammary bodies or stria terminalis causing a single "irritative" release of LHRF not observed with habenulum or lateral amygdal lesions (*752*). Testosterone propionate is the most potent of the sterilizing androgens given to the infantile rat, as is estradiol benzoate among the estrogens; various synthetic progestins and cortisol and cortisone had no sterilizing effect at relatively high dose, but progesterone at high dose was weakly effective (*753*). Doses of testosterone propionate markedly active in female infant rats do not impair spermatogenesis in infant male recipients, but androgen production appears much diminished (*754*). Ovulation in early life (at 10 weeks) with sterilization appearing later (at 13 to 21 weeks) is seen with low doses of testosterone propionate (*755*).

In adult female rats, sterilization may be accomplished by high doses (10–30 mg) of androgens such as dehydroisoandrosterone and androstenedione due to the induced formation of cystic ovaries (*756*) which outlast the inciting injection. Testosterone propionate implanted directly into the ovaries of hypophysectomized rats will stimulate antrum development and preserve corpora lutea, whereas its systemic administration is gonadotropin-inhibiting (*757*). Of course all of the naturally occurring androgens including the 11-hydroxylated adrenal products will, at appropriate dose, act as antigonadotropins [*244* (Ch. 4)] and may even directly inhibit uterine ova and embryos (*758*). Although a number of very active anti-androgens have been reported in recent years (cf. *759–761*), their effects on fertility in males or females remain to be elucidated.

The Activities of Gestagens

With the emergence of oral progestins as significant agents in fertility control, studies of their biological activities continue to multiply. In addition the synthesis and properties of new gestagens are the subject of multiplying publication. In Chapter 4 we have listed a good number of the newer compounds, particularly in relation to their ovulation-inhibiting activities. We have pointed out that there is no necessary correlation between their ovulation-inhibiting or antigonadotropic potencies and their progestational action. Nonetheless, the definition of their progestational activities is essential to the understanding of their roles in the regulation of reproductive processes. A true progestin may be defined as a compound which acts upon the uterus to induce endometrial proliferation and myometrial activity characteristic of pregnancy and which maintains pregnancy in ovariectomized animals carrying fertilized ova or fetuses; both of these functions may be enhanced by the concomitant use of small amounts of estrogen, but the progestin alone should be sufficient at adequate dose.

We early appreciated that in the new synthetic oral progestins even these two basic activities could be dissociated [*234* (Ch. 4)] since neither norethynodrel nor norethindrone maintained pregnancy in the rabbit though they readily induced pseudopregnant proliferation of the uterus. Drill and Riegel (*762*) recognized this dissociation and illuminated it further by reporting on the relative potency of a series of 17-alkyl-19-norsteroids in the test of McGinty *et al.* (*763*) involving local application to the rabbit uterine endometrium and in the systemic test of Clauberg [*609* (Ch. 7)]. In Table 28 we present their data on these two tests. It is obvious that a number of compounds inactive in the McGinty assay are quite active in the Clauberg test, e.g., II, VII. The reverse is less likely although V, highly active in the McGinty assay, is a poor oral progestin. In Table 29 several of the compounds of Table 28 are listed with their activity as maintainers of pregnancy [cf. *304* (Ch. 4)]. Norethynodrel (XVII), which is a poor endometrial progestin by subcutaneous administration but fairly active by the oral route, does not maintain pregnancy even when administered per os. One of the deductions made from this series is that the compounds inactive in the McGinty assay must be transformed to progestationally active compounds *in vivo*. Thus far in a search for the metabolites of norethynodrel in rabbit bile, urine, and feces we have not found a likely transformation product (*764*). Further studies are being made with C^{14}-labeled 19-norsteroids of this type. It will be noted that compound VIII is not included in Table 29. Tests in the rabbit indicate it to be fairly potent as a maintainer

TABLE 28

PROGESTATIONAL ACTIVITY[a] OF 19-NORTESTOSTERONE DERIVATIVES[b]
AND SOME 5(10)-ESTRENONE DERIVATIVES

Compound no.	Substituents	McGinty test (%)	Clauberg test	
			Subcutaneous (%)	Oral (%)
	19-Nortestosterone derivatives			
I	None	<0.5	<5	<20
II	17-Methyl	<0.5	500	100
III	17-Ethyl	25	500	250
IV	17-Propyl	500	250	25
V	17-Butyl	1000	100	<25
VI	17-Octyl	50	5–10	—
VII	17-Vinyl	<0.5	500	250
VIII	17-Ethynyl	<0.5	50	100
IX	17-Allyl	50	1000	250
X	17α-(1-Methallyl)	1000	500	50
XI	17-Methyldihydro	<0.5	10	<10
XII	17-Ethyldihydro	50	25	10
XIII	17-Propyldihydro	<0.5	<5	—
	5(10)-Estrenone derivatives			
XIV	17-Methyl	<0.5	5	25
XV	17-Ethyl	25–50	10–25	25 or >
XVI	17-Vinyl	<0.5	25	—
XVII	17-Ethynyl	<0.5	0–25	25
XVIII	17-Propyl	25	50	10

[a] Progesterone was assigned a potency of 100% and used as a standard.
[b] From Drill and Reigel (762).

of pregnancy when administered by injection, but with little or no activity per os [304 (Ch. 4)]. This would suggest a gut- or liver-engendered active metabolite.

Pregnancy maintenance by synthetic progestins in the rat has also been extensively studied [for a review of this and related assays see (765)]. Compounds II and III of Table 28 have 15 and

12 times, respectively, the activity of progesterone (required at 5 mg/day), 6-methyl-17-acetoxyprogesterone has 25 times the activity of progesterone and allylestrenol (the 3-deoxy derivative of compound IX) but 3 times the activity of progesterone on subcutaneous administration (766). Certain compounds required added estrogen to be effective, e.g., 1,2α-methylene-6-chloro-17α-acetoxy-Δ⁶-progesterone, 1000 parts to 1 of estradiol, or 17α-caproate-19-nortestosterone, 3000:1. Allylestrenol effectively maintains preg-

TABLE 29

PROGESTATIONAL ACTIVITY AND MAINTENANCE OF PREGNANCY IN RABBITS[a]

Compound no.	Compound	McGinty test (%)	Clauberg test, subcutaneous (%)	Maintenance of pregnancy (1 mg/kg)
	Progesterone[b]	100	100	89%
II	17-Methylnortestosterone	<0.5	500	0%
III	17-Ethylnortestosterone	25	500	64%
IV	17-Propylnortestosterone	500	250	80%
X	17α-1-Methallylnortestosterone	1000	500	100%
XVII	17-Ethynyl-Δ⁵⁽¹⁰⁾-nortestosterone	<0.5	0–25	0%
XVII	17-Ethynyl-Δ⁵⁽¹⁰⁾-nortestosterone		10–100 (oral)	0%

[a] From Drill and Riegel (762).
[b] Used as standard; assigned progestational potency in McGinty and Clauberg tests = 100%.

nancy in the ovariectomized rabbit with no interference even at large dose with the total transport of ova (767). In contrast, the 3-deoxy derivative of compound VIII, called lynestrol, will not maintain pregnancy in the rat despite oral endometrial progestational activity in the rabbit; in addition this compound fails to maintain deciduoma in mice; it acts as an ovulation inhibitor, a weak estrogen, and a weak androgen in rats (768).

The maintenance of pregnancy by progestins involves also a potency for prolonging normal pregnancy and preventing the induction of labor. The experimental prolongation in most test animals even for a few days usually leads to fetal death (769, 770). An interesting exception is the guinea pig which requires progesterone for maintenance only from the twelfth to twenty-first day, and thereafter to delivery neither ovaries nor exogenous hormone is required (*771*); in turn, there is no prolongation of pregnancy when either progesterone or synthetic gestagen is administered at the end of gestation (*772*). Norethindrone, which fails to support pregnancy in ovariectomized rabbits, will, at high dose, cause fetal death and prolongation of corpora lutea (*773*); thus its effect may be through stimulation of LTH production rather than via a direct effect on the uterus. A similar explanation may apply to the medroxyprogesterone-induced pregnancy prolongation accompanied by fetal mortality in ewes (*774*). However, in the inhibition of labor induced by oxytocin in the rabbit, medroxyprogesterone (MAP) is 10 to 100 times as active as progesterone, whereas 17-methyl-19-nortestosterone and allylestrenol are ineffective, although the latter will certainly prolong pregnancy at fairly high dose [*658* (Ch. 7)].

The progestational activity of a number of the compounds listed in Table 6 have been recently described in detail by Kincl and Folch Pi (*775, 776*). The compound most active by injection was 19-norprogesterone, and $6\alpha,16\alpha$-dimethyl-17-acetoxyprogesterone was most active by mouth. The potency of 3-deoxy steroids (e.g., ethylestrenol, lynestrenol) was much greater by the oral route than by injection, again suggesting a transformation product as the active agent. Among the newer progestational compounds reported in recent years we include: (a) various 6-substituted 6-dehydro-17-alkylprogesterones among which the 6-methyl compound has 130 and the 6-chloro compound 190 times the activity of 17-acetoxyprogesterone (*777*); (b) several dioxyprogesterones (*778*), among which 4-hydroxyl-17-acetoxyprogesterone is not only the most potent by Clauberg assay, but is also active in the McGinty test and maintains pregnancy in the rat when administered either by mouth or injection (*779*); (c) the acetophenone and acetonide derivatives of $16\alpha,17\alpha$-dihydroxyprogesterone, which are effective maintainers of pregnancy in the rat ovariectomized on day 8 (*780*), and the 2-acetofuran derivative of the $16\alpha,17\alpha$-dihydroxyprogesterone (*781*), which is a remarkably active depot progestin in the rabbit lacking androgenic, estrogenic, glucocorticoid, or fetal-virilizing activity; (d) various 16-alkylated progesterones (*782*); (e) 6-chloro-16-methyl- and 6-methyl-16-chloroprogesterones which are potent anti-estrogens as well as progestins (783); (f) various 21-carbon, 2-oxasteroids which are potent progestins (784); (g) 3-halo, Δ^5-pregnenes which are active despite the absence of α,β-unsaturation (785); (h) 21-halogenated derivatives of ethynyltestosterone and 19-nortestosterone and $\Delta^{9,10}$-estrenolone (786), all with progestational and antigonadotropic potency greater than the nonhalogenated parent compounds; (i) 3,17-dihydroxy-17α-ethynyl-19-nortestosterone-3,17-diacetate which is a weak estrogen, an extremely potent deciduomagenic compound, a good endometrial progestin, and ovulation inhibitor in the rabbit (787, 788); (j) some esters of 3β-hydroxy-4,6-dienes which retain activity of their parent 3-keto-Δ^4 progenitors (789); and (k) highly potent Δ^{11}-17-acetoxyprogesterone and some of its further unsaturated derivatives (790).

A number of effects of progestational steroids have been described which are significant but not directly related to gestational and antigestational functions. Thus the synchronization of estrous cycles in the ewe originally achieved by progesterone injection and withdrawal (791, 792) has been achieved by feeding and withdrawal of oral progestin in sheep (793, 794) and cattle (795). MAP and PMS will not only lead to highly fertile synchronized estrus but will bring up to 80% of anestrous ewes into heat with lambing in 50% of those bred (796). In domestic animals the 19-norsteroids have been used to inhibit nymphomania, control libido, and delay puberty (797). Control of estrus in the bitch by synthetic gestagens has also been described (798). Oral administration for one year of fairly low doses has been continuously effective in bitches and cats (799). The copulatory reflex in estrogen-primed guinea pigs which is induced by progesterone as well as other steroids (800) has been sought with a series of synthetic progestins (801); their effectiveness is not correlated with the usual measures of progestational activity. Indeed, testosterone-induced copulatory behavior in the guinea pig is inhibited by progesterone administration (802), but synthetic progestins have not been assayed.

Intrasplenic ovarian grafts in the guinea pig will hypertrophy apparently in response to endogenous gonadotropin. Suppression of this hypertrophy by gestagens may be used as a measure of their antigonadotropic potency. Withdrawal of the gestagen results in a rebound hypertrophy (*803*). Similarly the compensatory hypertrophy of the ovary remaining after hemiovariectomy has been examined as a measure of the antigonadotropic activity of the natural estrogens (estradiol, estrone, and estriol) and of various gestagens. The estrogens and norethynodrel (MED of 18–96 μg) will at higher dose stimulate ovarian growth and luteal development. They are more active than progesterone (MED 3630 μg), testosterone (MED 436 μg), norethisterone (MED 479 μg), or nobolethone (MED 155 μg), which at higher doses further depress ovarian weight, inhibit luteal development, and tend to increase the number of large vesicular and cystic follicles (*804*).

Although progesterone administration causes an increase in the total blood content of the rabbit uterus (*805*), the growth of *Escherichia coli* in the lumen is increased apparently because leucocytic infiltration is inhibited [99 (Ch. 2)]. An interesting effect of progesterone is its induction of a remarkable increase in incorporation of administered S^{35} by guinea pig cervical mucus (*806*). This presumably reflects the increase of sulfated mucopolysaccharides, perhaps chondroitin sulfuric acid. In the rabbit, progesterone administered alone induces a low columnar epithelium in the uterus, whereas progesterone with estrogen leads to a high columnar epithelium (*807*). Various synthetic gestagens act as if they were an estrogen-progestin combination (e.g., norethynodrel, ethynodiol acetate). In the golden hamster, a "decidual" endometrium is induced by norethandrolone and 11-deoxycorticosterone but not by an anabolic steroid or cortisone (*808*). Miyake *et al.* (*809*) have developed the deciduomagenic response of the estrogen-primed ovariectomized mouse as a means of quantitative assay for synthetic progestins, MAP and chlormadinone proving 2 to 14 times as active as progesterone, whereas norethindrone, norethynodrel, and 17-ethynyl testosterone were inactive. Indeed both local and systemic administration of these two 19-norsteroids and of estradiol led to an inhibition of the deciduomagenic action of progesterone. Two 5α-pregnanediols (20α and 20β) were inhibitory on local administration but not after parenteral administration.

Nor is the well-known growth-stimulating effect of progesterone on mammary glands imitated by all of the synthetic progestins. Using mammary DNA in estrogen-primed, ovariectomized rats as

an index of such stimulation, Griffith *et al.* (*810*) found no activity
exhibited by norethindrone or its 17-acetate in oral doses up to 2.7
mg per day, but they found excellent stimulation with 1 mg per
day of chlormadinone or MAP. Norethynodrel injected alone or
in combination with mestranol (as Enovid) into adult virgin rats
markedly stimulated lobule-alveolar mammary development to the
point of secretion (*811*). This may be attributable to stimulation of
the secretion of endogenous lactogenic hormone. In mice suckling
young, the administration of 17-hydroxyprogesterone caproate
(Delalutin) appeared to cause diminished milk production since the
young failed to gain weight at the normal rate (*812*). However, it
should be noted that Griffith *et al.* (*810*) observed an appetite
inhibition marked by weight loss in their progestin-fed animals, and
reduction in food consumption was observed in a 2-year toxicity
test with Orthonovum, which is norethindrone plus mestranol
(*813*).

A number of effects of progesterone are known to lie outside
of the reproductive process sphere. Increase of adrenal ascorbic
acid in progesterone-treated rats has been reported (*814*), suggesting inhibition of ACTH release or action, whereas norethynodrel
has been reported an inhibitor of the effects of cortisone acetate
upon rat adrenals, suggesting ACTH release or facilitation of its
action (*815*). In rats an inhibition of stress-induced release of
ACTH and the induction of adrenal atrophy by 6α-methyl-17-
acetoxyprogesterone have been reported (*816*), but the atrophied
adrenals will respond to ACTH administration (*817*). Furthermore,
the adrenal atrophy seen in rats [cf. *297* (Ch. 4)], rabbits, and
chickens (*818*) appears to be reversible, and was not observed
in mice or guinea pigs (*817*). In the latter animals a dosage effect
appears to be involved since others have observed in guinea pigs
receiving MAP (1 or 3 mg/kg/day) for 60 days a marked adrenal
atrophy with very low adrenal alkaline phosphatase activity; at the
low dose a restoration occurred by 30 days after discontinuance
but a persistance of relative atrophy was seen at this time in the
animals which had received the higher dose (*819*). Since progesterone is an adrenal precursor in the biosynthesis of corticosteroids it is not surprising to find evidence that an active adrenal
gestagen may be secreted. Thus Yamashita has found that the
administration of 4,4'-methylenedianiline increases endometrial car-

bonic anhydrase in the rabbit (*820*). This effect is blocked by cortisol administration and cannot be obtained in adrenalectomized animals, suggesting that inhibition of the normal course of steroidogenesis leads to gestagen production (*821*). Since 11-deoxycorticosterone maintains pregnancy in adrenalectomized rats (*822*), it as well as progesterone might be the gestagen. A direct effect of progesterone on the adrenal secretion of aldosterone has been noted in hypophysectomized rats (*823*). It appears to be quite specific since corticosterone secretion is unaffected in the same animals.

A diuretic effect of progesterone in the hypophysectomized rat (*824*), its hemopoietic action (*825*), its effects on hair growth (*826*) and maternal behavior (*827, 828*), its antiarrhythmic action on rat atria (*829*), its anti-bilharzia activity (*830*), and its stimulation of galactose metabolism (*831*) have not as yet been sought in the synthetics. Effects of Enovid upon blood vessel pattern in rabbits (*832*) and on ear vessel thrombosis in male hamsters (*833*) appear to have rather complex origins, and further study with this and other preparations seems to be needed.

Mention should be made of the effects of the discontinuance of use of gestagens. In rats made anovulatory by progesterone a withdrawal ovulation occurs regularly; it is not so easily inhibited by barbiturates and morphine as is normal, cyclic ovulation (*834*). The high plasma LH preceding this type of withdrawal ovulation may also be a feature in norethindrone acetate- and norethynodrel-blocked rats since the latter exhibit a marked increase in ova ovulated in the first postmedication ovulation (*835*) and the former a prompt fertility (*836*). In progesterone-suppressed goats the ova fertilized at the withdrawal ovulation have been transplanted to foster mothers with no indication of abnormal development (*837*). After pellet implantation of 19-norprogesterone for 395 days mice exhibit normal fertility despite the presence of ovarian tumors in some of these treated females (*838*).

Effects on Fetuses

Since a number of the synthetic progestins are derivatives of the androgens testosterone and 19-nortestosterone, their androgenic actions and particularly their potential for masculinizing female fetuses have been much studied. The usual test subject has been the post-implantation, pregnant rat injected for several days. The young at birth are usually examined for alteration in the anogenital separation (*839*). Actually inspection of the sex organs as well should be practiced (*840*). Indeed, only by such verification has detection been made of the virilizing action of allylestrenol (*841*); brief administration of large doses have allegedly led only to Wolffian duct persistence (*842*). Even with the use of strict criteria true virilization of rat fetuses has been claimed (*843*) and observed only in varying anogenital distance alterations (*844, 845*). Curiously, all groups of investigators are in complete agreement concerning the virilizing action of 6α-methyl-17-acetoxyprogesterone which may also cause fetal resorption in rabbits (*846*). Gestagenic compounds allegedly not virilizing to the rat fetus include chlormadinone (*844, 845*), the acetophenone and 3-acetofurane derivatives of 16α,17α-dihydroxyprogesterone (*843, 781*), 4-hydroxy-17-acetoxyprogesterone (*778*), 6-dehydroretroprogesterone (*847*), and 17-hydroxyprogesterone caproate (*848*). In contrast to chlormadinone its 1:2α-methylene derivative has an antimasculinizing effect on rat fetuses (*849*), and the irreversible underdeveloped genitalia appear to result from a competitive action on androgen receptors and not to any estrogenic or pituitary inhibiting effect of this powerful progestin (*850*). No progestin tested (progesterone, norethynodrel, and medroxyprogesterone) has affected the fetal mortality, malformations, and growth retardation induced by uterine vascular clamping in the rat (*851*). In mice, Turner *et al.* (*852*) find progesterone administration in a single large dose (50 mg) on day 11 will cause some clitoral enlargement and increase in anogenital distance in female fetuses; this tends to disappear with time. In contrast, testosterone proprionate in a single dose of 2 mg is markedly masculinizing to female fetuses. Possible differential mortality of male and female fetuses is suggested by the issue of 44% males in post-implantation ovariectomized pregnant rats maintained by progesterone plus estrogen and the issue of 55% males from intact, pregnant rats receiving the same steroid administration (*853*). Progesterone has indeed been shown to be directly toxic to mouse fetuses, but no sex difference has been reported (*854*).

Effects of nonsteroidal agents include: (a) complete sterilization of all fetuses of rats injected during pregnancy with busulfan (855) with a suggestion that premeiotic oogonia are special targets, and (b) many fetal abnormalities induced by 5-hydroxytryptamine administered to mice from days 5 to 12 of pregnancy (856). A review (857) of drug-induced embryopathies includes the action of a number of fertility-affecting agents.

Hormones and Tumors

The role that fertility-affecting hormones play in the development of tumors and the course of their growth has been exhaustively reviewed in a book (858) and in a number of articles (cf. 859, 860). Any attempt even to summarize the very extensive literature on this subject would be scarcely pertinent to the subject matter of this book. Many steroids and nonsteroidal compounds having hormonal properties have been studied as carcinogens and/ or cocarcinogens (861). Anticarcinogenic effects of alterations in the hormonal state of experimental animals (862, 863) have been analyzed. The therapeutic action of a number of hormonal and synthetic steroids in developed cancer in animals (859, 860) has been the subject of a large screening program conducted by the Cancer Chemotherapy Service Center of the National Cancer Institute of the United States Public Health Service (858). We shall discuss this topic in relation to some clinical studies.

The Metabolism of Compounds Affecting Fertility

A consideration of the anabolism and catabolism of the hormones concerned with reproductive processes would take us far beyond the scope of this book. Nonetheless, the relevance of these processes to fertility control is often emphasized. We have already noted that a key precursor to all the steroid hormones, Δ^5-pregnenolone, is an excellent sustainer of testis function in hypophysectomized rats. Similarly, an interference with cholesterologenesis in the gonads should be reflected in the nature and quantity of hormonal steroids produced (see Fig. 5). Each step in the biosynthetic sequence eventuating in hormone production is mediated by specific enzyme systems, some of which have been shown to be labile to a number of inhibitors, poisons, and so on. The hormones which stimulate gametogenesis also stimulate gonadal steroidogenesis. The receptor sites for gonadotropins stimulating steroidogenesis may indeed be quite different from those involved in follicle growth and rupture. Thus in the rabbit the increase in ovarian vein blood of progesterone and its 20-hydroxy derivative which follows coitus or gonadotropin injection may be due to interstitial tissue stimulation (864) just as testes hormone production is primarily a Leydig cell function. In rabbits the steroidogenic response of the ovaries to LH, mating, or electrical stimulation of the hypothalamus or medial amygdela (865) is extremely rapid, and appears to have a lower threshold than the ovulatory response (866). The marked stimulus by FSH of follicle growth seen in prepubertal rabbits is not accompanied by a capacity to convert Δ^5-pregnenolone to progesterone and 20α-hydroxy-Δ^4-pregnen-3-one; LH is needed for progestational steroidogenesis (867).

These findings on factors in steroid anabolism in the rabbit have some counterparts in other species studied. In the cycling mouse, maximal progesterone blood concentration is attained at proestrus, indicating an interstitial as wall as a luteal source in the ovary (868). The ovaries of prepuberal or hypophysectomized rats require FSH and LH for full functioning (869). A conversion of tritiated Δ^5-pregnenolone injected into the dog ovarian artery to 17-hydroxypregnenolone, progesterone, 17-hydroxyprogesterone, dehydroisoandrosterone, Δ^4-androstendione, testosterone, and estradiol has been reported to occur within 10 minutes (870). Ovarian vein progesterone in this species contains progesterone produced at a rate of 0.7 μg per ovary per minute which is unaffected by acute HCG administration but which increases 3- to 5-fold after several days injection of HCG or horse pituitary gonadotropin. Corpora lutea are responsible for the output since ovaries lacking corpora lutea yield little or no vein progesterone (871). In *Macacus* monkeys' ovary and blood, Hayward *et al.* (872) have observed HCG-induced increases in progesterone, in its 20-hydroxy derivative, and in 17α-hydroxyprogesterone in the absence of corpora lutea. In the mare, Short (873) finds in the follicular fluid estrogen (estrone, estradiol, 16-hydroxyestradiol), androgen (Δ^4-androstenedione, epitestosterone, 19-norandrostenedione), and progestin (progesterone, 17-hydroxyprogesterone); from the corpora lutea he has identified only 21-carbon steroid (progesterone, its 20α-hydroxy derivative, and a little 17-hydroxyprogesterone), indicating the absence of 17-desmolase in the luteal tissue. From bovine corpora lutea a soluble cholesterol sidechain cleaving enzyme system has been isolated which responds to FSH, LH, and HCG (*874*). It is TPNH-dependent and its activity may be inhibited by Δ⁵-pregnenolone or excess cholesterol (*875*). For progesteronogenesis a sensitivity of bovine corpora lutea to 10^{-10} molar LH concentration with FSH responsivity demanding a 100-fold increase in concentration suggests an exclusive dependence on LH since the FSH used was contaminated (perhaps to 1%) with LH (*876*). Again the progesteronogenic processes *may* proceed without corpora lutea since bovine fetal ovaries are able to perform the entire steroidogenic process from cholesterol to estrogen (*877*). The involuting corpus luteum in the cow loses its capacity to produce progesterone as the result of the unavailability of precursor (e.g., Δ⁵-pregnenolone) and the decline in cellular TPNH-generating capacity (*878*). An excellent review of steroidogenesis by corpora lutea by Savard *et al.* (*879*) summarizes both the biosynthetic transformations and the enzyme dependencies involved. A similar review of androgenesis (*880*) emphasizes species similarities in the biotransformations in all steroidogenic tissues.

The foregoing description of steroidogenic mechanisms and some of their dependencies illustrates briefly the complex chemical mechanisms underlying the production of the all-important sex hormones. Abnormalities in these mechanisms lead to sterility and aberrant sex functioning. Since they occur in males and females with, for the most part, only quantitative differences, both sexes may respond to imposed alterations in these mechanisms. Thus a common source of infertility might be the specific inhibition of 17-hydroxyprogesterone desmolase, leading to an overproduction of progestins and an underproduction of androgen and estrogen. This has been accomplished *in vivo* by diethylstilbestrol administration to mice (*881*) and *in vitro* by an indenyl pyridine (*882*); or an inhibition of 19-hydroxylation, e.g., by metopirone (*883*), might cause a relative overproduction of androgen and an underproduction of estrogen. The possibilities are as numerous as the specific biosynthetic steps and their essential components. What applies to steroidogenesis applies also to the genesis of the gonadotropins, of which we are all too ignorant.

Hormone catabolic processes similarly involve us in numerous potential disturbances of normal reproductive functioning. Perhaps one of the greatest safeguards to such normalcy is the extremely well-regulated set of hormone degradation mechanisms. The brief half-life of most hormones in the blood is a result of the operation of a dynamic equilibrating system (884, 885), the operation of which is better known theoretically than experimentally. Alterations in the rate of metabolic transformation or degradation of hormonal steroids may, in some measure, account for alterations in fertility. Thus the oral potency of some of the gestagens may be due to their ability to withstand liver degradative processes, and Cooke and Vallance (886) have indeed observed that in vitro rat and rabbit liver homogenates act more rapidly upon progesterone than on its 6α-methyl, its 17-acetoxy, or its Δ^6-6-methyl-17-acetoxy derivatives. Similarly, the superior potency of certain steroid enol ethers may be accountable to their relative resistance to degradative enzyme systems (887). The 17-alkylated gestagens are apparently protected from enzymic attack at carbon 17 since in rat liver homogenates in vitro the 17α-methyl group is retained unaltered although ring A reduction is rapidly accomplished (888). We have observed that the 17α-ethynyl group of norethindrone and norethynodrel are unchanged following parenteral administration to rabbits (764). The degree of lipoid solubility of a hormonal steroid may have a significant effect on its metabolism and action. From the rat gut the rate of absorption of steroids is greatest with those which are more lipoidal and least polar. The rate of absorption varies inversely with the extent of oxygenation (889). Storage of estrogen and androgen in body fat has long been known to affect apparent excretion rates (cf. 890), and the amount of progesterone stored has been found to vary with the stage of the estrous cycle (891). The stage of the cycle also appears to affect rates of progesterone conversion since in rats the ratio of progesterone to its 20-hydroxy derivative varies significantly (892). Adrenal steroid metabolites may affect reproductive activity, since marked adrenal stimulation by ACTH in mice inhibits ovarian maturation perhaps due to adrenal estrogen (*893*). An inhibitory effect of adrenal androgens upon the responsivity of mouse ovaries to PMS-HCG administration has been reported (*894*). We have already indicated that gestagens have no significant effect on ovarian responsivity to exogenous gonadotropins (cf. *895*), but a thorough study of their metabolites administered by various routes remains to be made.

The inactivation of gonadotropic hormones has not been examined to any great extent. Generally their inactivation may occur in their target organs (*896, 897*), but Dasgupta *et al.* (*898*) have observed active degradation *in vitro* of rat pituitary gonadotropin by rat liver, but not by spleen, diaphragm, or ovary. The damage of the liver by CCl_4 administration prevents liver inactivation. Thyroidectomy increases the inactivating capacity of the liver, and thyroxine administered either *in vitro* or *in vivo* inhibits inactivation.

When we consider that alterations may be made in the tissues and cells in which the regulatory hormones are metabolized, in their storage depots, and in the channels available for their excretion (i.e., urine, feces, sweat, milk), the normal maintenance of adequate functioning takes on an aura of improbability. In large measure the margins of safety in terms of turnover rates, critical concentrations, and compensatory feedbacks are remarkably wide. We long ago noted that steroid excretion rates vary manyfold in normal, healthy men and women and that individual output rates are characteristic and presumably reflective of rather constant endogenous production and/or degradation rates (*899*). A genetic determinant is suggested and the relationship of this to fertility would be worth examining.

REFERENCES

662. Cutting, W. 1962. *Stanford Med. Bull.* **20**, 152.
663. Ladman, A. J., and Soper, E. H. 1963. *Anat. Record* **145**, 332.
664. Applezweig, N. 1962. "Steroid Drugs." McGraw-Hill, New York.
665. Pincus, G. 1956. *In* "Currents in Biochemical Research" (D. Green, ed.), p. 176. Wiley (Interscience), New York.
666. Stone, G. M., and Martin, L. 1964. *Steroids* 3, 699.
667. Levitz, M., Money, W. L., Katz, J., and Dancis, J. 1964. *Endocrinology* **74**, 949.
668. Pincus, G. 1937. *Cold Spring Harbor Symp. Quant. Biol.* 5, 44.
669. Engel, L. L. 1961. *In* "Mechanism of Action of Steroid Hormones" (C. A. Villee and L. L. Engel, eds.), p. 1. Pergamon Press, New York.

670. Gordon, E. E., and Villee, C. A. 1956. *Endocrinology* **58**, 150.
671. Emmens, C. W. 1962. *In* "Methods in Hormone Research" (R. I. Dorfman, ed.), Vol. II, p. 59. Academic Press, New York.
672. Biddulph, C., Meyer, R. K., and Gumbreck, E. G. 1940. *Endocrinology* **26**, 280.
673. Genet, P., Henry, R., Vandel, S., Desfosses, B., and Jayle, M. F. 1962. *Ann. Endocrinol.* **23**, 693.
674. Velardo, J. T. 1958. *In* "The Endocrinology of Reproduction" (J. T. Velardo, ed.), p. 101. Oxford Univ. Press, London and New York.
675. Falconi, G. 1962. *Endocrinology* **71**, 657.
676. Pincus, G. 1950. *In* "The Hormones" (G. Pincus and K. Thimann, eds.), Vol. I, p. 333. Academic Press, New York.
677. Huggins, C., and Jensen, E. V. 1955. *J. Exptl. Med.* **102**, 335.
678. Velardo, J. T. 1959. *Ann. N. Y. Acad. Sci.* **75**, 441.
679. Leathem, J. H. 1959. *Ann. N. Y. Acad. Sci.* **75**, 463.
680. Chu, E. W., Wurtman, R. J., and Axelrod, J. 1964. *Endocrinology* **75**, 238.
681. Wurtman, R. J., Axelrod, J., Chu, E. W., and Fischer, J. F. 1964. *Endocrinology* **75**, 266.
682. Săhleanu, V., Holban, R., Janivă, E., and Serban, A. M. D. 1963. *Commun. Acad. Rep. Populare Romine* **13**, 141.
683. Bever, A. T. 1959. *Ann. N. Y. Acad. Sci.* **75**, 472.
684. Villee, C. A. 1961. *In* "Sex and Internal Secretions" (W. C. Young, ed.), Vol. I, p. 643. Williams & Wilkins, Baltimore, Maryland.
685. Mueller, G. C., Herranen, A. M., and Jervell, K. F. 1958. *Recent Progr. Hormone Res.* **14**, 95.
686. Hayashi, M., and Fishman, W. H. 1961. *Acta Endocrinol.* **38**, 107.
687. Bo, J. W. 1959. *J. Histochem. Cytochem.* **7**, 403.
688. Harris, R., and Cohen, S. 1951. *Endocrinology* **48**, 264.
689. Wallace, J. C., Stone, G. M., and White, I. G. 1964. *J. Endocrinol.* **29**, 175.
690. Lammes, F. B., and Willighagen, G. J. 1963. *Nature* **98**, 394.
691. Jensen, E. V., and Jacobson, H. I. 1960. *In* "Biological Activities of Steroids in Relation to Cancer" (G. Pincus and E. Vollmer, eds.), p. 161. Academic Press, New York.
692. Bengtsson, G., and Ulberg, S. 1963. *Acta Endocrinol.* **43**, 561.
693. Bengtsson, G., and Ulberg, S. 1963. *Acta Endocrinol.* **43**, 581.
694. Stone, G. M. 1964. *J. Endocrinol.* **29**, 127.
695. Martin, L., and Baggett, B. 1964. *J. Endocrinol.* **30**, 41.
696. Hechter, O., and Lester, G. 1960. *Recent Progr. Hormone Research* **16**, 139.
697. Villee, C. A., and Engel, L. L., eds. 1961. "Mechanism of Action of Steroid Hormones." Pergamon Press, New York.
698. Hechter, O., and Halkerston, I. D. K. 1964. *In* "The Hormones" (G. Pincus, K. Thimann, and E. Astwood, eds.), Vol. 5, p. 697. Academic Press, New York.

699. Karlson, P. 1961. *Deut. Med. Wochschr.* **86**, 663.
700. Zalokar, M. 1961. *In* "Control Mechanisms in Cellular Processes" (D. M. Bonner, ed.), p. 87. Ronald Press, New York.
701. Hechter, O., and Halkerston, I. D. K. 1965. *Ann. Rev. Physiol.* **27**, 133.
702. Gorski, J. 1964. *J. Biol. Chem.* **239**, 889.
703. Segal, S. J. 1964. *Anat. Record* **148**, 334.
704. Wilson, J. D. 1963. *Proc. Natl. Acad. Sci. U. S.* **50**, 93.
705. Mueller, G. C., Gorski, J., and Aizawa, Y. 1961. *Proc. Natl. Acad. Sci. U. S.* **47**, 164.
706. Ui, H., and Mueller, G. C. 1963. *Proc. Natl. Acad. Sci. U. S.* **50**, 256.
707. Noteboom, W. D., and Gorski, J. 1963. *Proc. Natl. Acad. Sci. U. S.* **50**, 250.
708. Szego, C. M., and Roberts, S. 1953. *Recent Progr. Hormone Res.* **8**, 419.
709. Nicolette, J. A., and Gorski, J. 1964. *Endocrinology* **74**, 955.
710. Dorfman, R. I. 1961. *In* "Mechanism of Action of Steroid Hormones" (C. A. Villee, and L. L. Engel, eds.), p. 148. Pergamon Press, New York.
711. Fishman, W. H. 1961. *In* "Mechanism of Action of Steroid Hormones" (C. A. Villee, and L. L. Engel, eds.), p. 157. Pergamon Press, New York.
712. Villee, C. A., Hagerman, D. D., and Joel, P. B. 1960. *Recent Progr. Hormone Res.* **16**, 49.
713. Szego, C. M., and Sloan, S. H. 1961. *Gen. Comp. Endocrinol.* **1**, 295.
714. Rudzik, A. D., and Miller, J. W. 1962. *J. Pharmacol. Exptl. Therap.* **138**, 88.
715. Wurtman, R. J., Axelrod, J., and Potter, L. T. 1964. *J. Pharm. Exptl. Therap.* **144**, 150.
716. Iversen, O. H. 1962. *Acta Pathol. Microbiol. Scand.* **56**, 245.
717. Fowler, D. D., Szego, C. M., and Glasser, S. R. 1963. *Endocrinology* **72**, 701.
718. Cecil, H. C., Bitman, J., and Wrenn, T. R. 1964. *Endocrinology* **74**, 701.
719. Dorfman, R. I., and Kincl, F. A. 1963. *Steroids* **1**, 185.
720. Dorfman, R. I., ed. 1962. "Methods in Hormone Research," Vol. II, p. 113. Academic Press, New York.
721. Loken, B., Uskokovic, M., Hagopian, M., Dorfman, R. I., and Gut, M. 1963. *Steroids* **2**, 81.
722. Hecker, E., and Farthofer, G. 1963. *Biochim. Biophys. Acta* **71**, 196.
723. Edgren, R. A., Weinberg, I. P., and Cochran, T. G. B. 1963. *Endocrinology* **72**, 665.
724. Lee, A. E., and Williams, P. C. 1964. *J. Endocrinol.* **28**, 199.
725. Kraus, S. D. 1962. *Proc. Soc. Exptl. Biol. Med.* **109**, 78.
726. Sonnen, N., Goldhauser, R., and Carson, S. 1962. *Endocrinology* **71**, 779.
727. Goldhauser, R., Sonnen, N., and Carson, S. 1962. *Federation Proc.* **21**, 388.
728. Adler, J. H. 1962. *Vet. Record* **74**, 1148.
729. Leavitt, W. W., and Wright, P. A. 1963. *J. Reprod. Fertility* **6**, 115.

730. Cook, H., and Kitts, W. D. 1964. *Acta Endocrinol.* **45**, 33.
731. Szego, C. M., and Sloan, S. H. 1963. *Endocrinology* **72**, 626.
732. Christian, J. J. 1962. *Federation Proc.* **22**, 507.
733. Spaziani, E. 1962. *Proc. Soc. Exptl. Biol. Med.* **111**, 637.
734. Costăchel, O., Zinca, V., Dănicel, M., and Popp, I. 1961. *Acad. Rep. Populare Romine Inst. Endocrinol. Prof. C. I. Parhon Studii Cercetari Endocrinol.* **12**, 791.
735. Nicola, A. A., Lantos, C. P., and Tramazzani, J. H. 1962. *Experientia* **18**, 467.
736. Kitay, J. I. 1963. *Endocrinology* **73**, 253.
737. Heim, L. M., and Timiras, P. S. 1963. *Endocrinology* **72**, 598.
738. Wilson, J. G., Young, W. C., and Hamilton, J. B. 1940. *Yale J. Biol. Med.* **13**, 189.
739. Pfeiffer, C. A. 1936. *Am. J. Anat.* **58**, 195.
740. Young, W. C. 1961. *In* "Sex and Internal Secretions" (W. C. Young, ed.), Vol. II, p. 1173. Williams & Wilkins, Baltimore, Maryland.
741. Whalen, R. E., and Nadler, R. D. 1963. *Science* **141**, 273.
742. Kikuijania, S. 1963. *Annotationes Zool. Japon.* **36**, 145.
743. Gorski, R. A. 1963. *Am. J. Physiol.* **205**, 842.
744. Harris, G. W. 1964. *Proc. 7th Conf. Intern. Planned Parenthood, Singapore* p. 478. Excerpta Medica, Amsterdam.
745. Gorski, R. A., and Wagner, J. W. 1964. *Anat. Record* **148**, 373.
746. Kincl, F. A., Folch Pi, A., and Herrera-Lasso, L. 1963. *Endocrinology* **72**, 966.
747. Barraclough, C. A. 1961. *Endocrinology* **68**, 62.
748. Harris, G. W. 1963. *J. Reprod. Fertility* **5**, 299.
749. Gorski, R. A., and Barraclough, C. A. 1962. *Acta Endocrinol.* **39**, 13.
750. Brown-Grant, K., Quinn, D. L., and Zarrow, M. X. 1964. *Endocrinology* **74**, 811.
751. Johnson, D. C., and Witschi, E. 1963. *Endocrinology* **73**, 467.
752. Hagino, N., Wagner, J. W., and Gorski, R. A. 1964. *Anat. Record* **148**, 288.
753. Gorski, R. A. 1963. *Anat. Record* **145**, 234.
754. Swanson, H. E., and Van der Werff ten Bosch, J. J. 1963. *J. Endocrinol.* **26**, 197.
755. Swanson, H. E., and Van der Werff ten Bosch, J. J. 1964. *Acta Endocrinol.* **45**, 1.
756. Ron, S., Mahesh, V. B., and Greenblatt, R. B. 1962. *Nature* **196**, 42.
757. Igel, H. 1962. *Zentr. Gynaekol.* **84**, 1227.
758. Meyer, C. J., Krahenbuhl, C., and Desaulles, P. A. 1963. *Acta Endocrinol.* **43**, 27.
759. Lerner, L. J., Bianchi, A., and Borman, A. 1960. *Cancer* **13**, 1201.
760. Dorfman, R. I., Fajkos, J., and Joska, J. 1964. *Steroids* **3**, 675.
761. Saunders, H. L., Holden, K., and Kerwin, J. F. 1964. *Steroids* **3**, 687.

762. Drill, V. A., and Riegel, B. 1958. *Recent Progr. Hormone Res.* 14, 29.
763. McGinty, D. A., Anderson, L. P., and McCullagh, N. B. 1939. *Endocrinology* 24, 829.
764. Arai, K., Golab, T., Layne, D. S., and Pincus, G. 1962. *Endocrinology* 71, 639.
765. Junkmann, K. 1963. *Deut. Med. Wochschr.* 88, 629.
766. Suchowsky, G. K. 1963. *Acta Endocrinol.* 42, 533.
767. Wu, D. H. 1962. *Endocrinol. Japon.* 9, 187.
768. Overbeek, G. A., Madjerek, Z., and de Visser, J. 1962. *Acta Endocrinol.* 41, 351.
769. Nelson, W. P., Pfiffner, J. J., and Haterins, H. O. 1930. *Am. J. Physiol.* 91, 690.
770. Moore, H. C. 1963. *J. Obstet. Gynaecol. Brit. Commonwealth* 70, 151.
771. Deansley, R. 1963. *J. Reprod. Fertility* 6, 143.
772. Zarrow, M. X., Anderson, N., and Gallantine, M. 1963. *Nature* 198, 690.
773. Huiming, W. D. 1961. *T'ai-wan I Hsueh. Hui Tsa Chih* 60, 23.
774. Bengtsson, L. P., and Schofield, B. M. 1963. *J. Reprod. Fertility* 5, 423.
775. Kincl, F. A., and Folch Pi, A. 1962. *Ciencia (Mex.)* 22, 35.
776. Kincl, F. A., and Folch Pi, A. 1962. *Ciencia (Mex.)* 22, 31.
777. Weiss, M. J., Schaub, R. E., Poletto, J. F., Allen, G. R., Jr., and Pidacks, C. C. 1963. *Steroids* 1, 608.
778. Arcari, G., Baldratti, G., and Sala, G. 1963. *Nature* 197, 292.
779. Baldratti, G., and Sala, G. 1962. *Acta Endocrinol.* 40, 113.
780. Lerner, L. J., Brennan, D. M., Yiacas, E., De Phillipo, M., and Borman, A. 1962. *Endocrinology* 70, 283.
781. Lerner, L. J., Yiacas, E., and Borman, A. 1963. *Proc. Soc. Exptl. Biol. Med.* 113, 663.
782. Shapiro, E., Legatt, F., Weber, L., Steinberg, M., Watnick, A., Eisler, M., Hennessey, M. G., Corriglio, C. T., Charney, W., and Oliveto, E. P. 1962. *J. Med. Pharm. Chem.* 5, 975.
783. Rapula, R. T., and Murray, M. J., Jr. 1962. *J. Med. Pharm. Chem.* 5, 1049.
784. Pappo, R., and Jung, C. J. 1962. *Tetrahedron Letters* 9, 365.
785. Halpern, O., Edwards, J. A., and Zderick, J. A. 1962. *Chem. & Ind. (London)* p. 1571.
786. Steelman, S. L., Morgan, E. R., and Busch, R. D. 1962. *Federation Proc.* 21, 213.
787. Elton, R. L., Nutting, E. F., and Saunders, F. J. 1962. *Acta Endocrinol.* 41, 381.
788. Drill, V. A. 1963. *J. Reprod. Fertility* 5, 462.
789. Baran, J. S. 1963. *J. Med. Chem.* 6, 329.
790. Dusza, J. P., Joseph, J. P., Heller, M., and Bernstein, S. 1963. *J. Med. Chem.* 6, 364.
791. Robinson, T. J. 1956. *Australian J. Agr. Res.* 7, 194.

792. Lamond, D. R. 1962. *Proc. Australian Soc. Animal Prod.* 4, 72.
793. Evans, J. S., Dutt, R. H., and Simpson, E. C. 1962. *J. Animal Sci.* 21, 804.
794. Southcott, W. H., Braden, A. W. H., and Moule, G. R. 1962. *Australian J. Agr. Res.* 13, 901.
795. Van Blake, H., Brunner, M. A., and Hansel, W. 1963. *J. Dairy Sci.* 46, 459.
796. Brunner, M. A., Hansel, W., and Hogue, D. E. 1964. *J. Animal Sci.* 23, 32.
797. Jöchle, W., Merkt, H., Rüsse, M., Schilling, E., Smidt, D., and Zerobin, K. 1964. *J. Endocrinol.* 29, i.
798. Cameron, R. S. 1962. *Vet. Record* 74, 1136.
799. Huris, T. W., and Wolchuk, N. 1963. *Am. J. Vet. Res.* 24, 1003.
800. Boling, J. L., Young, W. C., and Dempsey, E. W. 1938. *Endocrinology* 23, 182.
801. Kincl, F. A., and Dorfman, R. I. 1961. *Acta Endocrinol.* 38, 257.
802. Diamond, M., and Young, W. C. 1963. *Endocrinology* 72, 429.
803. Haller, J. 1963. *J. Reprod. Fertility* 5, 297.
804. Peterson, D. L., Edgren, R. A., and Jones, R. C. 1964. *J. Endocrinol.* 29, 255.
805. Kao, C. Y., and Gam, R. S. 1961. *Am. J. Physiol.* 201, 214.
806. Gothie, S. 1961. *Pathol. Biol. Semaine Hop.* 9, 655.
807. Elton, R. L. 1962. *Anat. Record* 142, 469.
808. Czyba, J. C., and Chiris, M. 1963. *Compt. Rend. Soc. Biol.* 157, 1587.
809. Miyake, T., Kakushi, H., and Hara, K. 1963. *Steroids* 2, 749.
810. Griffith, D. R., Williams, R., and Turner, C. W. 1963. *Proc. Soc. Exptl. Biol. Med.* 113, 401.
811. Kahn, R. H. 1964. *Anat. Record* 148, 296.
812. Mazza, A., Russo, R., and Hecht-Lucari, G. 1963. *Monit. Ostetrico-ginecol.* 34, 266.
813. King, T. O., and Lubansky, F. 1962. *Pharmacologist* 4, 176.
814. Jakowicki, J. 1961. *Endokrynol. Polska* 12, 487.
815. Mazza, A., Cascialli, M., Diversi, F., Barbieri, M., and Hecht-Lucari, G. 1962. *Ostet. Ginecol.* 33, 379.
816. Holab, D. A., Katz, F. H., and Jailer, J. W. 1961. *Endocrinology* 68, 173.
817. Arends, J. 1963. *Arch. Pharm. Chemi* 70, 907.
818. Schomberg, D. W., Stob, M., and Andrews, F. N. 1964. *Gen. Comp. Endocrinol.* 4, 54.
819. Coletta, A., Frigeri, E., and Persico, M. 1963. *Ostet. Ginecol.* 68, 94.
820. Yamashita, K. 1963. *Nature* 200, 81.
821. Yamashita, K. 1963. *Am. J. Physiol.* 205, 195.
822. Anderson, R. R., and Turner, C. W. 1963. *Am. J. Physiol.* 205, 1077.
823. Singer, B., Losito, C., and Salmon, S. 1963. *J. Endocrinol.* 28, 65.
824. Selye, H., and Bassett, L. 1940. *Proc. Soc. Exptl. Biol. Med.* 44, 502.
825. Vollmer, E. P., and Gordon, A. S. 1941. *Endocrinology* 29, 828.

826. Dannecl, R., and Kallo, L. 1947. Z. *Naturforsch.* **2b**, 215.
827. Riddle, O., Lahr, E. L., and Bates, R. W. 1936. *Yearbook Carnegie Inst.* **35**, 49.
828. Koller, G. 1952. *Verhandl. Deut. Zool. Ges.* p. 160.
829. Gimeno, A. L., Gimeno, M., and Webb, J. L. 1963. *Calif. Med.* **98**, 67.
830. Lagrange, E. 1963. *Compt. Rend. Soc. Biol.* **157**, 425.
831. Topper, Y. J., Maxwell, E. S., and Pesch, L. A. 1960. *Biochim. Biophys. Acta* **37**, 563.
832. Danforth, D. N., Manalo-Estrella, P., and Buckingham, J. C. 1964. *Am. J. Obstet. Gynecol.* **88**, 952.
833. Sichuk, G., Bettigole, R. E., Fortner, J. G., and Rawson, R. W. 1964. *Federation Proc.* **23**, 412.
834. Hoffman, J. C., and Schwartz, N. B. 1964. *Federation Proc.* **23**, 109.
835. Lakshman, A. B., and Nelson, W. O. 1963. *Nature* **199**, 608.
836. Iturriza, F. C., and Restelli, M. A. 1963. *Semana Med. (Buenos Aires)* **122**, 1285.
837. Nishikawa, Y., Horie, T., Sugie, T., Onuma, H., and Niwa, T. 1963. *Proc. Japan Acad.* **39**, 758.
838. Lipschutz, A., Iglesias, R., and Salinas, S. 1963. *J. Reprod. Fertility* **6**, 99.
839. Suchowsky, G. K., and Junkmann, K. 1961. *Endocrinology* **68**, 341.
840. Schoeler, H. F. L., and de Wachter, A. M. 1961. *Acta Endocrinol.* **38**, 128.
841. Jost, A., and Moreau, M. G. 1963. *Compt. Rend. Acad. Sci.* **256**, 502.
842. Mey, R. 1963. *Acta Endocrinol.* **44**, 27.
843. Lerner, L. J., De Phillipo, M., Yiacas, E., Brennan, D. M., and Borman, A. 1962. *Endocrinology* **71**, 448.
844. Kincl, F. A., and Dorfman, R. I. 1962. *Acta Endocrinol.* **41**, 274.
845. Kraay, R. J., and Brennan, D. M. 1963. *Acta Endocrinol.* **43**, 412.
846. Mey, R. 1963. *Geburtsh. Frauenheilk.* **23**, 291.
847. Jost, A. 1963. *Acta Endocrinol.* **43**, 539.
848. Johnstone, E. E., and Franklin, R. K. 1964. *Obstet. Gynecol.* **23**, 359.
849. Hamada, H., Neumann, F., and Junkmann, K. 1963. *Acta Endocrinol.* **44**, 380.
850. Junkmann, K., and Neumann, F. 1964. *Acta Endocrinol. Suppl.* **90**, 139.
851. Franklin, J. B., Goldfarb, A. F., Matsumoto, R., and Brent, J. L. 1963. *Fertility Sterility* **14**, 365.
852. Turner, C. D., Asakawa, H., and Lin, H. S. 1964. *Am. Zool.* **4**, 289.
853. Hahn, E. W., and Hays, R. L. 1963. *J. Reprod. Fertility* **6**, 409.
854. Petrelli, E. A., and Forbes, T. R. 1964. *Endocrinology* **75**, 145.
855. Hemsworth, B. N., and Jackson, H. 1953. *J. Reprod. Fertility* **6**, 229.
856. Paulson, E., Robson, J. M., and Sullivan, F. M. 1963. *J. Endocrinol.* **26**, xxv.
857. Fave, A. 1964. *Thérapie* **1**, 1.

858. Pincus, G., and Vollmer, E. P., eds. 1960. "Biological Activities of Steroids in Relation to Cancer." Academic Press, New York.
859. Muhlbock, O. 1962. *In* "The Morphological Precursors of Cancer" (E. Severi, ed.). Perugia, Div. Cancer Res.
860. Noble, R. L. 1964. *In* "The Hormones" (G. Pincus, K. Thimann, and E. B. Astwood, eds.), Vol. V, p. 559. Academic Press, New York.
861. Huggins, C. 1963. *J. Am. Med. Assoc.* **186**, 481.
862. Glucksmann, A., and Cherry, C. P. 1962. *Brit. J. Cancer* **16**, 634.
863. Talwalker, P. K., Meites, J., and Mizuno, H. 1964. *Proc. Soc. Exptl. Biol. Med.* **116**, 533.
864. Hilliard, J., Archibald, D., and Sawyer, C. H. 1963. *Endocrinology* **72**, 59.
865. Hilliard, J., Hayward, J. N., and Archibald, D. 1963. *Anat. Record* **145**, 239.
866. Hilliard, J., Hayward, J. N., and Sawyer, C. H. 1964. *Anat. Record* **148**, 291.
867. Endroczi, E., Hayward, J. N., Hilliard, J., and Sawyer, C. H. 1964. *Federation Proc.* **23**, 109.
868. Guttenberg, I. 1961. *Endocrinology* **68**, 1006.
869. Ahren, K., and Kostyo, J. L. 1963. *Endocrinology* **73**, 81.
870. Aakvaag, A., and Eik-Nes, K. B. 1964. *Biochim. Biophys. Acta* **86**, 380.
871. Romanoff, E. B., Deshpande, N., and Pincus, G. 1962. *Endocrinology* **70**, 532.
872. Hayward, J. N., Hilliard, J., and Sawyer, C. H. 1963. *Proc. Soc. Exptl. Biol. Med.* **113**, 256.
873. Short, R. V. 1962. *J. Endocrinol.* **24**, 59.
874. Ichii, S., Forchielli, E., and Dorfman, R. I. 1963. *Steroids* **2**, 631.
875. Toren, D., Menon, K. M. J., Forchielli, E., and Dorfman, R. I. 1964. *Steroids* **3**, 381.
876. Mason, N. R., and Savard, K. 1964. *Endocrinology* **74**, 664.
877. Roberts, J. D., and Warren, J. C. 1964. *Endocrinology* **74**, 846.
878. Armstrong, D. T., Black, D. L., and Cone, C. E. 1964. *Federation Proc.* **23**, 462.
879. Savard, K., Marsh, J. M., and Rice, B. F. 1965. *Recent Progr. Hormone Res.* **21**. (In press.)
880. Dorfman, R. I., Forchielli, E., and Gut, M. 1963. *Recent Progr. Hormone Res.* **19**, 251.
881. Samuels, L. T., Short, J. G., and Huseby, R. A. 1964. *Acta Endocrinol.* **45**, 487.
882. Hall, P. F., Eik-Nes, K. B., and Samuels, L. T. 1963. *Endocrinology* **73**, 547.
883. Griffiths, K. 1963. *J. Endocrinol.* **26**, 445.
884. Van de Wiele, R. L., MacDonald, P. C., Gurpide, E., and Lieberman, S. 1963. *Recent Progr. Hormone Res.* **19**, 275.
885. Tait, J. F. 1963. *J. Clin. Endocrinol. Metab.* **23**, 1285.

886. Cooke, B. A., and Vallance, D. K. 1964. *Biochem. J.* **90**, 31P.
887. Ercoli, A. 1962. *Proc. 1st Intern. Congr. Hormonal Steroids,* p. 6. Excerpta Medica, Amsterdam.
888. Hiraji, O., Kichisaburo, M., and Tokuda, G. 1964. *Acta Endocrinol.* **46**, 40.
889. Schedl, H. P., and Clifton, J. A. 1961. *Gastroenterology* **41**, 491.
890. Takaheshi, K. 1961. *Tohoku J. Appl. Med.* **75**, 207.
891. McCracken, J. A. 1964. *J. Endocrinol.* **28**, 339.
892. Eto, T., Masuda, H., Suzuki, Z., and Hoshi, F. 1962. *Japan. J. Animal Reprod.* **8**, 34.
893. Christian, J. J. 1964. *Endocrinology* **74**, 669.
894. Varon, H. H., and Christian, J. J. 1963. *Endocrinology* **72**, 210.
895. Smith, B. D., and Bradbury, J. T. 1964. *Anat. Record* **148**, 337.
896. Wijnans, M. 1954. *Acta Physiol. Pharmacol. Neerl.* **3**, 199.
897. Sgouris, J. T., and Meites, J. 1952. *Am. J. Physiol.* **169**, 301.
898. Dasgupta, P. R., Kar, A. B., and Das, C. 1964. *Proc. Soc. Exptl. Biol. Med.* **116**, 253.
899. Pincus, G., Romanoff, L. P., and Carlo, J. 1954. *J. Gerontol.* **9**, 113.

III
CLINICAL STUDIES

CHAPTER 9

Control of Fertility in Men

The natural history of the human male is such that the development of infertility is often considered a pathological phenomenon, even in elderly men. The clear demonstration of testicular sperm in about 50% of men in their ninth and tenth decades (900) suggests that the loss of spermatogenetic capacity need not be as inevitable as the loss of ovogenetic and ovulating potency. Nonetheless, with advancing age, increasing fibrosis, hyalinization of the connective tissue, and arteriolar arteriosclerosis tend to be the rule (901, 902). An increase in Sertoli cell glycogen and especially lipid accumulation is observed (903) along with hypertrophy of immature spermatogenic cells and a relative loss of spermatids (904). A decrease in size and number of Leydig cells has been associated with decreased potency and libido. However, a lack of correlation between clinical symptoms, androgen levels as judged by urinary excretion and testicular cytology (905), leads one to suspect that psychogenic and other unknown factors obscure the syndrome called the male climacteric. Reporting on a study of testicular biopsies and hormone excretion of almost 100 men ranging in age from 60 to 94, Segal and Nelson (906) conclude that 15% have testicular function not unlike that of much younger men. Ten percent showed regression of testicular function and high gonadotropin excretion. About 5% had genuine testis atrophy secondary to hypophyseal impairment. In over 50%, functional Leydig cells were obvious, but with a tendency to estrogen predominance in their secretory activity. We noted some time ago that certain urinary estrogens show a relative increase in advancing age and total estrogen certainly does increase

187

relative to total androgen (*907*). Recently the development of accurate methods for the measurement of plasma and urinary testosterone, the "true" testis androgen, may offer an opportunity for more meaningful functional correlations (*908, 909*).

Many of the studies of the aging testis have been made with men suffering from prostatic carcinoma since palliative therapy in such cases involves castration with the removal of at least superficially healthy testes (*910*). According to Sommers (*911*), prostatic cancer cases have a pituitary cytology reflective of the action of excess estrogen which may be of adrenal origin in castrates. Alternate and complementary treatment is high dose estrogen administration. We therefore have numerous accounts of estrogen effects upon the human testis (cf. *912, 913*). The admirable summary by Albert [*34* (Ch. 2)] is: "Estrogen induces atrophy of the tubules and the Leydig cells; the latter revert to fibroblasts. The germinal epithelium shows an increase in lipids and a decrease in glycogen. Unless other disease is present the atrophy proceeds so that only the Sertoli cells remain in the tubules; even these cells may disappear with the induction of peritubular hyalinization and sclerosis." This remarkable sterilizing action of estrogen has not been put to use for contraceptive purposes; an obvious objection is the induction of impotence and of gynecomastia with the use of sterilizing doses. The recent use of relatively low doses of estrogen as well as of impeded estrogens in men with myocardial infarcts (*914, 915*) should offer an opportunity for further determinations of effects in the sexual sphere.

On the basis of certain clinical syndromes there was postulated a number of years ago a human testicular hormone designated as inhibin (*916*). Its function was primarily to inhibit pituitary gonadotropic output. The experimental evidence for and against the inhibin hypothesis has been reviewed by Albert [*34* (Ch. 2)], with the conclusion that the evidence for the production of such a hormone is inadequate. Estrogen secretion by the human testes may indeed explain the clinical findings (*917*). Recently Johnson (*918*) in a detailed study of urinary gonadotropin, androgen metabolism, and germinal epithelium changes in various hypogonadal men has come to the conclusion that a testis-secreted inhibin offers the only logical explanation of the data obtained.

The effect of androgen administered to men has also been the subject of much inquiry. Its chief value has been in the treatment of hypogonadal states, but studies have been made of its use in many other conditions. In Table 30, taken from Dorfman and Shipley (919), are listed the various therapeutic studies made with androgens and the deductions made therefrom. Perhaps the most notable is the use in oligospermia. Actually androgen administered to men with normal testes ordinarily depresses the sperm count (920) with depression of the germinal epithelium and concomitant inhibition of urinary gonadotropin output (921). In men with oligospermia and inadequate spermatogenesis, testosterone proprionate administration further accentuates testis dysfunction with tubular necrosis, hyalinization, and disappearance of Leydig cells. On withdrawal of treatment, a "rebound" occurs in about 50% of such cases with increase of sperm count and improvement in tubular appearance (922, 923). Albert [34 (Ch. 2)] avers that the rebound phenomenon is transient at best and may even be adventitious. Noting increased urinary estrogenic activity in men receiving testosterone and remarking on the estrogen-like effect upon the testis of androgen administration, Paulsen (924) has attributed the suppressive effect on gonadotropin output to the presumed estrogen metabolite of testosterone. Breuer (925) has observed a small (0.02% to 0.07%) yield of estrogens in the urine of men receiving testosterone, its 19-nor derivative or of androsta-1,4-diene-3,17-dione.

The first use of oral ovulation-inhibiting progestin in men treated daily for up to 5 months with Enovid was reported in 1957 (926). Sterilizing action was clearly indicated in testicular biopsies which showed absence of spermatogenesis, ill-formed lumina with peritubular sclerosis, and reduction in Leydig cells. The estrogenic component of the medication may have been the agent responsible for these changes. However, later studies with a nonestrogenic progestin, 17α-ethyl-19-nortestosterone, by Heller and his associates (927) revealed many similar effects. Furthermore, in a number of gestagen-treated men, withdrawal led to a clear "rebound" with markedly increased sperm count (928) and complete tubular recovery. In further studies, Heller et al. (929) noted that the depression of sperm count by progesterone was not accompanied by alterations in either gonadotropin or estrogen excretion nor was there more

TABLE 30

SUMMARY OF CLINICAL USEFULNESS OF ANDROGEN THERAPY IN VARIOUS DISORDERS[a]

Positive indication. Response is invariably good	Response sometimes observed but element of suggestion undoubtedly is important	Response sometimes observed but primary disorder probably not effected. Nonspecific tonic effect is a factor	Usefulness not yet established or evidence conflicting although favorable effects reported	No clear-cut therapeutic effect yet established	Contraindicated
Response good in many cases and is probably due to a relatively direct hormonal effect					
Primary hypogonadism	Prostatism	Cushing's syndrome	Convalescence from chronic illness	Arteriosclerosis	Cancer of male breast
Hypogonadism of proved chronicity	Angina pectoris	Cirrhosis of liver	Premature infants	Nephrosis	Cancer of prostate
Male climacteric	Enuresis	Involutional melancholia	Gynecomastia	Nonhypogonadal impotence	
Undescended testes (gonadotropin treatment preferred)		Muscular dystrophy	Renal tubular necrosis	Homosexuality	
Pituitary dwarfism		Hyperthyroidism	Cholera		
Panhypopituitarism[b]			Simple senility		
Oligospermia[b]			Simple retardation of growth		
Adherent foreskin			Addison's disease (as supplementary therapy)		

[a] From Dorfman and Shipley (919).
[b] Rebound after cessation of therapy.

than slight tubal depression. In contrast, 17α-ethyl-19-nortestoster-
one (Nilevar) treatment revealed involution of all germinal elements without hyalinization of the basement membrane, urinary
gonadotropin suppression, and estrogen output increase. They
deduce that the last two compounds may be converted to estrogens
or be inherently "estrogenic" as pituitary gonadotropin suppressors,
that Nilevar acts directly as an antigonadotropin and that progesterone (in the dose used) has no pituitary depressing effect but
probably acts directly on the testis to suppress sperm production
by an unknown mechanism. Heller and Clermont (930) have
demonstrated that Nilevar at high dose causes a hypoplasia of the
seminiferous epithelium, inhibits the formation of spermatozoa,
and depresses the number of their precursors, but has no effect
on the rate of development of the germ cells which are still present
in the seminiferous epithelium. Since HCG administration similarly
failed to affect this rate, calculated as 74 days for the total course
of spermatogenesis (cf. 931), they concluded that the endogenous
seminiferous cycles in man are a biological invariant. Similar failure
to alter the rate of spermatogenesis by variations in endocrine states
has been reported for the ram (932) and the rat (933). Apostolokis
(934) examined the effects of norethisterone taken daily by oligo-
spermic men for periods varying from 25 to 70 days. Azoospermia
occurred in most cases and the reduction in sperm count was in
each case preceded by a drop in urinary gonadotropin. Urinary
corticosteroids, estrogens and, in most cases, 17-ketosteroids were
unaffected. Direct action of 17-methyl-19-nortestosterone upon the
testis does not appear to occur since its administration did not
inhibit HCG stimulation of the testis in men with testis hypo-
function (935).

Since libido and potency were reduced in these subjects by each
compound tested, their utility as antifertility agents has been questioned. As rather large doses were used (15 mg/day or more for
several months) the possibility of differential action on tubules
(such as seemed to occur with progesterone) at lower progestin
dose is suggested. Indeed, 6α-methyl-17-acetoxyprogesterone may
have such an effect even at moderate doses (936).

Limited investigation has been made of the effects of corticosteroids on testis function in men. The development of testicular
atrophy in men with Cushing's syndrome (937) has suggested an

antifertility effect of endogenous corticosteroid. However, no very marked derangement in testicular function were seen in arthritic men receiving large doses of cortisone (938); apparent stimulation of FSH secretion with no effect on LH secretion was observed [118 (Ch. 3)]. Prednisolone in doses of 20 to 30 mg per day for 21 days had no effect on ejaculate volume, sperm count, or seminal fructose. Larger doses, up to 250 mg per day for about 10 days, did markedly reduce ejaculate volume, sperm count, and seminal fructose (939).

Several of the nonsteroidal agents affecting spermatogenesis in male animals have been studied in men. Among them a potent nitrofuran derivative, nitrofurantoin, has been administered to men, and with therapeutic doses no significant effects on sperm production have been seen; unpleasant side effects marked the use of doses affecting spermatogenesis (940). Three of the bis(dichloroacetyl)amines found to be so effective in animals [152 (Ch. 3)] have been studied in human subjects by Heller and colleagues in volunteer prison inmates (941). Two of the three effectively reduced the sperm count to below 4 million per cc within 8 to 11 weeks. Combination of one with stilbestrol (0.1 mg/day) led to complete azoospermia in several subjects. No effects of any drug (or the combination with stilbestrol) inhibited Leydig cell function as judged by testicular biopsy and urinary steroid output; nor was pituitary inhibition indicated by gonadotropin excretion assays. The suppressive action on spermatogeneis proved to be reversible. Minor gastrointestinal side effects were noted. Testicular biopsies from volunteer users (942) reveal only minor effects on spermatogenesis. As with the steroid hormones, there is no effect on the duration of the cycle. The major effects appeared to be a decrease in the total number of spermatids and nuclear and acrosomal abnormalities in maturing spermatids. Leydig cells appeared to be normal but a rise in urinary gonadotropin secretion suggests the possibility of a reduced production of testis steroid normally inhibitory to high gonadotropin output. The spermatozoa in the ejaculate of users exhibited the abnormalities described for the maturing spermatids (943), and a slow return to normal morphology and motility followed cessation of use.

Nelson (944) has confirmed these observations, but found that individuals ingesting these drugs experience an exaggerated response to the peripheral effects of alcohol. The marked severe cardiovascular and CNS system effects suggest interference with the metabolic degradation of alcohol (*945*). These alarmingly unpleasant, but not serious, reactions make acceptability unlikely.

Experimental studies of sperm (or testes) antibodies in men have not been very extensive. The antigenicity of human testes and sperm has, of course, been well established [*179* (Ch. 3), *946*]. Auto-antibodies have been found to occur spontaneously as sperm agglutinins in the serum of men. According to Rümke and Hellinga (*947*) such agglutinins are found in 1% of normal fertile men and in 4.1% of 2000 sterile men examined. Nelson (*944*) reports briefly of preliminary adjuvant-aided testis immunization studies in volunteer subjects by Mancini. Davidson (*948*) has observed aspermatogenesis in men receiving injections of autologous and homologous testes in Freund's adjuvant. Sloughed germinal epithelium was observed in biopsies after 45 days of injection, and at 5 months more advanced lesions were present. The presence of sperm and seminal plasma agglutinins has been studied by Southam (*949*) in fertile and sterile couples. Demonstrated fertility in many of these subjects (as in the agglutinin-produced fertile males examined by Rümke and Hellinga) suggests that antibodies with sterilizing action are unlikely. Perhaps of more than passing interest are as yet unidentified but nonetheless effective intravaginal spermicidal factors observed in certain infertile matings (*950*).

The vulnerability of scrotal testes to a damaging effect of heat upon the spermatogenetic process has long been known for a number of mammalian species. The extensive tubular degeneration and testis damage has been noted in a previous chapter. In a recent review (*951*) of the experimental data with animals a report has been given of unpublished experiments of Tokuyama. Taking cognizance of the observation that in men whole body exposure in fever therapy cabinets produces a significant drop in sperm counts at 3 to 7 weeks after the exposure (*952*), Tokuyama studied 18 human volunteers aged 21 to 26 who accepted local heat application to the scrotum and its structures. A single exposure for 30 minutes at temperatures between 40°C and 47°C led to a significant drop in sperm counts 5 to 7 weeks later. Depression of sperm counts to extremely low levels was obtained by repeated exposures, and the low counts could be maintained by one application every 3 weeks but not by one every 4 weeks.

It is obvious from the foregoing that experimental studies with men have been quite limited. This has been in part due to a relative paucity of leads from animal studies. Generally men have come to experimental observation because of sterility problems and major concerns have been with the sperm count and factors affecting it, coital frequency, libido, fertility and so on [cf. 56 (Ch. 2), 953, 954]. In spite of excellent quantitative measures of male fertility in sperm count and seminal fructose (cf. 955) and the clear indications of seminiferous epithelium and Leydig cell function to be had from testis biopsies (956, 957), male volunteers for fertility control studies may be numbered in the low hundreds whereas women have volunteered for similar studies by the thousands. Actually the human male with the use of the condom is by far the predominant practitioner of contraception. Apparently, however, he has psychological aversions to experimenting with sexual functions. In countries where vasectomy and abortion are equally available, the latter practice overwhelmingly exceeds the former, e.g., Japan. Indeed, sterilization in Japan occurs in women with about 20 times the frequency that it does in men (958) despite the fact that in women a major and in men a minor surgical procedure is involved. Perhaps experimental studies of fertility control in men should be preceded by a thorough investigation of male attitudes.

REFERENCES

900. Belonoschkin, B. 1954. *Fertility Sterility* 5, 182.
901. Engle, E. T. 1955. *Recent Progr. Hormone Res.* 11, 291.
902. Leathem, J. H. 1958. *In* "The Endocrinology of Reproduction" (J. T. Velardo, ed.), p. 315. Oxford Univ. Press, London and New York.
903. Lynch, K. M., and Scott, W. W. 1950. *J. Urol.* 64, 767.
904. Mellgren, J. 1945. *Acta Pathol. Microbiol. Scand. Suppl.* 60, 1.
905. Goldzieher, J. W., and Hamblen, E. C. 1947. *Surg., Gynecol. Obstet.* 85, 583.
906. Segal, S. J., and Nelson, W. O. 1959. *In* "Endocrinology of Reproduction" (C. W. Lloyd, ed.), p. 107. Academic Press, New York.
907. Pincus, G. 1961. *In* "Growth in Living Systems" (M. X. Zarrow, ed.), p. 407. Basic Books, New York.

908. Dorfman, R. I. 1962. *In* "Methods in Hormone Research" (R. I. Dorfman, ed.), Vol. 1, p. 51. Academic Press, New York.
909. Riondel, A., Tait, J. F., Gut, M., Tait, S. A. S., Joachim, E., and Little, B. 1963. *J. Clin. Endocrinol. Metab.* **23**, 620.
910. Huggins, C. 1946. *J. Am. Med. Assoc.* **131**, 576.
911. Sommers, S. C. 1957. *Cancer* **10**, 345.
912. Schwartz, M. 1945. *Proc. Am. Federation Clin. Res.* **2**, 97.
913. de la Balze, F. A., Gurturden, A. I., Janches, M., Arillaga, F., Alvarez, A. S., and Segal, L. 1962. *J. Clin. Endocrinol.* **22**, 1251.
914. Pincus, G., ed. 1959. "Hormones and Atherosclerosis." Academic Press, New York.
915. Marmorston, J., Moore, F. J., Hopkins, C. E., Kuzuma, O. T., and Weiner, J. 1962. *Proc. Soc. Exptl. Biol. Med.* **110**, 400.
916. Klinefelter, H. F., Jr., Reifenstein, E. C., Jr., and Albright, F. 1942. *J. Clin. Endocrinol.* **2**, 615.
917. Goldzieher, J. W., and Roberts, I. S. 1952. *J. Clin. Endocrinol.* **12**, 143.
918. Johnsen, S. G. 1964. *Acta Endocrinol. Suppl.* **90**, 99.
919. Dorfman, R. I., and Shipley, R. A. 1956. "Androgens." Wiley, New York.
920. Heckel, N. J. 1940. *J. Urol.* **43**, 286.
921. Heller, C. G., Nelson, W. O., and Roth, A. A. 1943. *J. Clin. Endocrinol.* **3**, 573.
922. Heller, C. G., Nelson, W. O., Maddock, W. O., Jungck, E. C., Paulsen, C. A., and Mortimer, G. E. 1951. *J. Clin. Invest.* **30**, 648.
923. Heckel, N. J., and McDonald, J. H. 1952. *Ann. N. Y. Acad. Sci.* **55**, 725.
924. Paulsen, C. A. 1952. *J. Clin. Endocrinol.* **12**, 915.
925. Breuer, H. 1962. *Acta Endocrinol.* **40**, 111.
926. Pincus, G. 1957. *In* "Proc. Symposium on 19-Nor Progestational Steroids," p. 105. G. D. Searle & Co., Chicago, Illinois.
927. Heller, C. G., Laidlaw, W. M., Harvey, H. T., and Nelson, W. O. 1958. *Ann. N. Y. Acad. Sci.* **71**, 649.
928. Heller, C. G., Moore, D. J., Paulsen, C. A., Nelson, W. O., and Laidlaw, W. M. 1959. *Federation Proc.* **18**, 1057.
929. Heller, C. G., Paulsen, C. A., and Moore, D. J. 1960. *Proc. 1st Intern. Congr. Endocrinol.* p. 925.
930. Heller, C. G., and Clermont, Y. 1964. *Recent Progr. Hormone Res.* **20**, 545.
931. Heller, C. G., and Clermont, Y. 1963. *Science* **140**, 184.
932. Ortavant, R. 1958. Thèse Ph.D. Faculté des Sciences, Université de Paris, Paris.
933. Harvey, S. C., and Clermont, Y. 1962. *Anat. Record* **142**, 239.
934. Apostolokis, M. 1961. *Acta Endocrinol.* **37**, 75.
935. Huis in't Veld, L. G., Louwerens, B., and van der Spek, P. A. F. 1961. *Acta Endocrinol.* **37**, 217.
936. MacLeod, J. 1965. *In* "Symposium on Agents Affecting Fertility." (In press.)

937. Heinbecker, P. 1944. *Medicine* **23**, 225.
938. McDonald, J. H., and Heckel, N. J. 1955. *Trans. Am. Assoc. Genito-Urinary Surg.* **44**, 6.
939. Weller, O. 1962. *Endokrinologie* **43**, 135.
940. Nelson, W. O., and Bunge, R. G. 1957. *J. Urol.* **77**, 275.
941. Heller, C. G., Moore, D. J., and Paulsen, C. A. 1961. *Toxicol. Appl. Pharmacol.* **3**, 1.
942. Heller, C. G., Flageolle, B. Y., and Matson, L. J. 1963. *Exptl. Mol. Pathol. Suppl.* **2**, 107.
943. MacLeod, J. 1961. *Anat. Record* **139**, 250.
944. Nelson, W. O. 1963. *Marriage and Family Living* **25**, 74.
945. Heller, C. G., and Moore, D. J. 1963. *Am. Chem. Soc. Div. Med. Chem. Abstr.*, p. 32L.
946. Katsh, S. 1963. *J. Reprod. Fertility* **5**, 290.
947. Rümke, P., and Hellinga, G. 1959. *Am. J. Clin. Pathol.* **32**, 357.
948. Davidson, O. W. 1962. *In* "Proceedings of a Conference on Immuno-Reproduction" (A. Tyler, ed.), p. 27. The Population Council, New York.
949. Southam, A. L. 1963. *J. Reprod. Fertility* **5**, 458.
950. Masters, W. H., and Johnson, V. E. 1961. *Fertility Sterility* **12**, 560.
951. Leblond, C. P., Steinberger, E., and Roosen-Runge, E. C. 1963. *In* "Mechanisms Concerned with Conception" (C. G. Hartman, ed.), p. 1. Macmillan, New York.
952. MacLeod, J., and Hotchkiss, R. S. 1941. *Endocrinology* **28**, 780.
953. Farris, E. J. 1951. *Brit. Med. J.* **II**, 1475.
954. Joel, C. A. 1960. *Fertility Sterility* **11**, 384.
955. Schirren, C. 1963. *J. Reprod. Fertility* **5**, 347.
956. Nelson, W. O., and Heller, C. G. 1948. *Recent Progr. Hormone Res.* **3**, 197.
957. Clermont, Y. 1963. *Am. J. Anat.* **112**, 35.
958. Koya, Y. 1963. "Pioneering in Family Planning." Japan Medical Publ., Tokyo, Japan.

CHAPTER 10

Fertility in Women—Ovogenesis and Ovulation

Fertility Potential in Women

Fertility in women depends upon the normal production, fertilization, tubal transport and cleavage, uterine entry, blastocyst development, and implantation of ova and the maintenance of the fetus to parturition. In reviewing the ontogeny of human ova, Hartman (959) has concluded: "the hazards of the human ovum from ovulation, fertilization and nidation to birth are the same fundamentally in the human species as in the rest of the Mammalia." Logically, then, the experimental studies concerned with female animals should find application in women and, indeed, most of them do. There are some variations in detail, but the basic controlling processes appear to be identical. The mystery of ovogenesis in women is exemplified by the count of from 100,000 to 1,000,000 oocytes in human infants' ovaries and the estimate that in 30 years of reproductive life a maximum of 390 of these ova are ovulated. Out of 34 human ova collected from the oviducts by Hertig, Rock, and Adams (960) within the first 17 days of development, 13 were palpably abnormal. Compared to the enormous oocyte loss this 40% wastage may seem less than trifling, but the practical implications are obviously important. When to this tentative rate of loss we add the less easily determined losses due to abortion [calculated as occurring spontaneously in up to 20% of all conceptions

TABLE 31

Classification of Endocrine Syndromes Associated with Pathologic Findings in the Ovary[a]

Hormone status	Syndrome	Clinicopathological findings	Associated ovarian pathology
Estrogen excess (or prolonged uninterrupted estrogen)	Estrinism: 1. Precocious puberty 2. Metropathia hemorrhagica (or other menstrual disorders) 3. Postmenopausal bleeding	Metrorrhagia, amenorrhea Enlargement of breasts, and secondary sex development Hyperplasia of endometrium (? carcinoma) and tubal epithelium Hypertrophy of myometrium (? myomas) Cornification of vaginal mucosa	Single follicle cysts Polycystic ovaries Granulosa-theca cell tumors Rare Sertoli-Leydig and lipoid cell tumors
Estrogen lack (or slight androgen excess)	Defeminization (or failure of feminization)	Oligomenorrhea, amenorrhea Breast atrophy and regression of secondary sex characteristics Atrophy of endometrium, myometrium, tubal epithelium, and vaginal mucosa	Ovarian atrophy (or agenesis) Polycystic ovaries Germinomas Masculinizing ovarian tumors
Androgen excess	Masculinization (with or without defeminization)	Hirsutism Enlargement of clitoris Temporal hair recession and baldness Enlargement of larynx and voice changes Masculine habitus	Polycystic ovaries with hyperthecosis Hilus cell hyperplasia Sertoli-Leydig cell tumors Lipoid cell tumors Rare granulosa-theca cell tumors
Corticosteroid excess	Cushing's syndrome (with or without masculinization)	Adiposity of trunk, striae Polycythemia Hypertension Diabetic tendency Osteoporosis	Lipoid cell tumors

[a] From Morris and Scully (962).

(*961*) depending in part on locality] and complications thereof a considerable wastage of fertility potential is obvious.

These spontaneous checks on fertility have relatively unknown etiology. It is common to ascribe many of them to genetic lethal factors. Among the proven limiting factors to normal ovum development in women we have: (a) the time of ovulation, (b) the frequency and timing of coitus, (c) the age of the ovum at the time of sperm penetration and (d) influences, including infections, on ovum transport and nidation. Less well analyzed are factors associated with the aging of sperm in the oviducts, nutritional, including avitaminoses and toxins, limitations to ovum development, utero-hypophyseal relationships, the receptivity of the aging uterus, and effects of psychic and physical stresses. However fascinating it might be to do so, it is beyond the province of this book to catalog the numerous pathological states and conditions that have been found to contribute to female sterility. The list is long and the putative interrelationships complex and difficult. For example, in considering the limited area of ovarian pathologies associated with endocrine syndromes we emerge with Table 31 taken from Morris and Scully (*962*). This table only presents associations with steroid hormone aberrations, probably because these have some ease of recognition. If we were to add to this other possible endocrine involvements, including pituitary pathologies, thyroid and parathyroid dysfunctions, and so on, a treatise of no mean dimensions might well emerge. What we propose considering here are the leads to and means of control of fertility in normal women of reproductive age.

Detection of Ovulation

The surest sign of ovulation is the establishment of a pregnancy. The early detection of pregnancy thus offers the first testimony to the significance of a missed menstruation. The basis for practically all pregnancy tests is the remarkable increase first observed by Aschheim and Zondek (*963*) in the excretion into urine of gonadotropin of chorionic origin (HCG). Until recently highly accurate diagnosis has been based on the responses of ovaries or testes of test animals. These tests have been thoroughly reviewed by Zarrow

[*81* (Ch. 2)] from whose article Table 32 is taken. The availability of highly purified HCG has led to its use as an antigen and the establishment of a pregnancy test based on a hemagglutination reaction (*969*) using pregnancy urine as the HCG source. Serum HCG in pregnant women may be assayed by hemagglutinin inhibition and also used for pregnancy diagnosis (*970.*) These immunoassay methods have received considerable testing (*971, 972*) and

TABLE 32
PREGNANCY TESTS WITH AN ACCURACY OF 98 TO 100%[a]

Animal	Sex	Observed end point	Time (hr)	Reference
Immature mouse	F	Corpora hemorrhagica	96	*964*
Isolated rabbit	F	Corpora hemorrhagica	48	*965*
Xenopus laevis	F	Extrusion of ova	8–12	*966*
Bufo arenarum	M	Extrusion of sperm	2–4	*967*
Immature rat	F	Hyperemia of ovary	4	*968*

[a] From Zarrow (*81*).

have been found to offer certain advantages over animal tests (*973*). The failure to induce vaginal bleeding within 15 hours following ingestion of a progestin-estrogen combination has also been studied as a pregnancy test (*974*). Although offering a 92% certainty in pregnancy, it may be misleading in women entering the menopause, in prolonged amenorrhea, and in women taking psychotropic drugs (*975*).

Obviously these pregnancy tests diagnose a fertile ovulation, but offer no means for the detection of the more usual cyclical ovulations. The various methods employed for this purpose have been exhaustively reviewed by Hartman (*959*). Those which do not involve direct observation of the ovaries or of eggs and embryos may be classified as inconstant (e.g., intermenstrual pain or bleeding, cervical mucus secretions) and regularly recurring, i.e., vaginal epithelium desquamation, endometrial changes, basal body temperature (BBT) alterations, and hormone excretions.

That the daily vaginal smear offers a routine means of determining the approximate time of ovulation was first demonstrated by Papanicolaou (*976*), and a somewhat more rapid method for smear staining designed particularly for ovulation diagnosis was described by Shorr (977). Ovulation time is marked by a predominating proportion of large, flat, well-dispersed, cornified cells and a minimum of leucocytes (978). Recently Hammond (979) has modified vaginal smear staining by the use of pyocyanole, and finds it rather sharply differentiates the smooth, pale cytoplasm of ovulatory stage cells from the heavily granular, curled or wrinkled post-ovulatory cells. Castellanos and Sturgis (980) find a parallel to the vaginal changes in the cytology of cells centrifuged down in urine samples. In the follicular phase, or under estrogen administration, 20% or more of the cells are cornified. In the luteal phase or during progestin administration the proportion of cornified cells is markedly reduced.

The sequence of endometrial changes reflecting the cyclical variations in ovarian hormone secretion was elaborately analyzed by Schröder (981), and subsequently confirmed by numerous observers. The preovulatory proliferative phase is followed beginning just after ovulation by a secretory phase which supervenes only in the presence of an active, progestin-secreting corpus luteum. Using day 14 as the most frequent ovulation time, the dating of the endometrium into 28-day stages has now become common practice; a 15-day endometrium marks the beginning of endometrium gland secretion, a 1-day endometrium the initiation of menstruation, and so on (982, 983).

Recording and analysis of the BBT has been denominated by Hartman (959) as the most practically applied criterion of ovulation in women. The typical biphasic curve with its temperature shift at approximately mid-cycle is now a gynecological commonplace. The rise from relatively low to relatively high temperature marks "ovulation time." A standard BBT curve is shown in Fig. 15. The low temperatures during the follicular phase are ascribed to the temperature-depressing activity of estrogen and the thermogenic action of progesterone has been held accountable for the luteal phase elevation. The most convincing evidence of this has been the data obtained following estrogen and progestion administration to ovariectomized women (984, 985). The wide variability in the temperature graph has been noted by many observers, but the consensus appears to be that "only rarely does one see a chart on which the apparent sign of ovulation is beyond the limits of 14 ± 4 days before the onset of flow" (986). In the study of almost 1100 cycle records from 155 healthy, fertile women, Marshall (987) finds 1% of anovulatory cycles and the temperature rise occurring most commonly at 13 days before the next period. Vollman (988) in a study of a series of single fertile copulations finds the optimal fertile time to precede the temperature rise by 2 days and the occurrence of cervical mucorrhea by 3 days. This accords well with

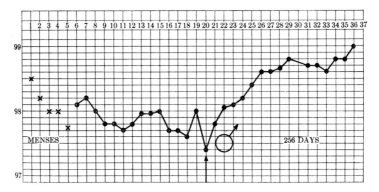

FIG. 15. A "classical" BBT curve. [After Hartman (959).]

similar data of Haman (989) and Pommerenke (990) who described data on isolated fertile coitus and successful artificial insemination in 134 and 159 cases, respectively. For an amusing account of the psychological basis of apparent ovulation times deduced from the testimony of wives of husbands on brief furlough during war and from alleged cases of rape the reader is referred to Chapter 24 of Hartman (959).

Just as pregnancy is the indubitable sign of a fertile ovulation, so is the rise in urinary pregnanediol during the menstrual cycle an unequivocal demonstration of the establishment of an active corpus luteum. This invaluable discovery of Venning and Browne (991) was based on the measurement of urinary pregnanediol glucuronide. Latterly pregnanediol derived by hydrolysis has been measured directly with somewhat greater ease and accuracy, but the basic findings of Venning and Browne remain, and are illustrated in Fig. 16 which demonstrates: (a) an initial appearance

centages in control and Enovid-using subjects' ovaries are identical in the several age groups and the mean oocyte density is indeed elevated in the older Enovid users (due to absence of large follicles). Despite the finding of elevated luteal phase urinary pregnanediol in some 6.8% of users of Orthonovum (10 mg) suggesting

TABLE 42

ATRESIA PERCENTAGES AND OOCYTE DENSITIES IN OVARIAN BIOPSIES
FROM ENOVID USERS AND CONTROL SUBJECTS

Age range (yr)	Control subjects			Enovid users		
	No.	% Atretic follicles	Follicles per mm²	No.	% Atretic follicles	Follicles per mm²
18–25	15	80 ± 3.3[b]	0.79 ± 0.13[b]	9	63 ± 8.0[b]	1.77 ± 0.75[b]
26–29	5	67 ± 8.7	0.39 ± 0.12	8	47 ± 8.2	1.78 ± 0.72
30–33	13	58 ± 6.8	0.38 ± 0.16	9	67 ± 9.0	0.31 ± 0.11
34–37	27	61 ± 4.6	0.22 ± 0.05	—	—	—
38–42	7	67 ± 4.5	0.09 ± 0.03	5	53 ± 7.3	0.31 ± 0.07[a]

[a] Underlined value significantly different from control value.
[b] ± standard error.

possible establishment of a corpus luteum (*1154*) ovulation prevention seems to offer the most satisfactory explanation of the mechanism of oral steroid contraception. Increased pregnanediol output due to adrenocortical stress reaction is a possible occasional event or even elevated thecal cell secretion in unovulated ovaries (cf. *1186*).

Inhibition of ovulation has also been attempted by the injection of depot progestins. This has been reported for 17-hydroxyprogesterone caproate (Delalutin) by Siegel (*1187*) who observed complete absence of conceptions in 25 postpartum women receiving 500 mg injections every 4 weeks on six successive occasions followed thereafter by 4 weekly intervals in which the progestin was administered in combination with estradiol valerate. Injection of medroxyprogesterone acetate as a depot ovulation inhibitor led to lengthened menstrual cycles and heavier menstrual flow (*1188*). Since this compound without estrogen appears to be a poor ovulation inhibitor (*1189*), the effects of its injection in combination with an estrogen will undoubtedly be reported.

The nonsteroidal inhibitor of ovulation, a dithiocarbamoxyl-hydrazine [133 (Ch. 3)], has been administered orally to postmenopausal women and in doses of 300 mg per day induced a decrease in urinary gonadotropin (1190). Administration of 50 mg per day to normally cyclic women led to a postponement of ovulation during its use (1191) and in some women approaching menopause a withdrawal menstruation (1192). Its cyclic use with added estrogen to induce regular cyclic menstruation may be possible (1193).

REFERENCES

1082. Pincus, G. 1955. Proc. 5th Intern. Conf. Planned Parenthood, Tokyo, Japan, p. 175.
1083. Pincus, G., Rock, J., and Garcia, C.-R. 1958. Ann. N. Y. Acad. Sci. 71, 677.
1084. Rock, J., Pincus, G., and Garcia, C.-R. 1956. Science 124, 891.
1085. Rock, J., Garcia, C.-R., and Pincus, G. 1957. Recent Progr. Hormone Res. 13, 323.
1086. Garcia, C.-R., Pincus, G., and Rock, J. 1958. Am. J. Obstet. Gynecol. 75, 82.
1087. Rice-Wray, E. 1957. In "Proceedings of the Symposium on 19-Norprogestational Steroids," p. 78. G. D. Searle & Co., Chicago, Illinois.
1088. Pincus, G., Rock, J., Garcia, C.-R., Rice-Wray, E., Paniagua, M., and Rodriguez, I. 1958. Am. J. Obstet. Gynecol. 75, 1333.
1089. Pincus, G., Garcia, C.-R., Rock, J., Paniagua, M., Pendleton, A., Laraque, F., Nicolas, R., Borno, R., and Pean, V. 1959. Science 130, 81.
1090. Pincus, G., Rock, J., and Garcia, C.-R. 1959. Proc. 6th Intern. Conf. Planned Parenthood, New Delhi, India p. 216.
1091. Pincus, G. 1961. "Modern Trends in Endocrinology," 2nd Series, p. 231. Butterworth, London.
1092. Guttmacher, A. F. 1962. Postgrad. Med. 32, 552.
1093. Jöchle, W. 1962. Angew. Chem. 1, 537.
1094. Richter, R. H. H., and Schreiner, W. E. 1963. Therap. Umschau 20, 489.
1095. Kaiser, R. 1963. Deut. Med. Wochschr. 88, 2325.
1096. Proc. 3rd Conf. for Europe, Near East, and Africa. Intern. Planned Parenthood Federation 1963. Excerpta Med. No. 71. Amsterdam, Holland.
1097. Tyler, E. T. 1964. J. Am. Med. Assoc. 187, 562.
1098. Berczeller, P. H., Young, I. S., and Kupperman, H. S. 1964. Clin. Pharmacol. Therap. 5, 216.
1099. Madsen, V. 1964. Ugeskrift Laeger 126, 95.
1100. Pincus, G., and Bialy, G. 1964. Advan. Pharmacol. 3, 285.

1101. Pincus, G. 1960. In "Clinical Endocrinology" (E. B. Astwood, ed.), Vol. I, p. 526. Grune & Stratton, New York.
1102. Rock, J. 1961. In "Control of Ovulation" (C. A. Villee, ed.), p. 222. Pergamon Press, New York.
1103. Nevinny-Stickel, J. 1963. Zentr. Gynaekol. 85, 865.
1104. Volkaer, R., and Kridelka, C. 1963. Ann. Endocrinol. 21, 49.
1105. Swyer, G. I. M., and Little, V. 1962. Proc. Roy. Soc. Med. 55, 861.
1106. Carter, W. F., Faucher, G. L., and Greenblatt, R. B. 1964. Am. J. Obstet. Gynecol. 89, 635.
1107. Mears, E. 1965. Symp. on Antifertility Agents. In press.
1108. Eckstein, P., Waterhouse, J. A. H., Bond, G. M., Mills, W. G., Sandilands, D. M., and Shotton, D. M. 1961. Brit. Med. J. II, 1172.
1109. Mears, E. 1963. Brit. Med. J. I, 1318.
1110. Swyer, G. I. M. 1964. Intern. J. Fertility 9, 11.
1111. Nevinny-Stickel, J. 1964. Intern. J. Fertility 9, 57.
1112. Haller, J. 1962. Acta Endocrinol. Suppl. 67, 131.
1113. Kitagawa, K., Hirata, M., and Tokuda, G. 1963. Matsushita Bull. Human Sci. 4, 10.
1114. Roland, M., Clyman, M. J., Decker, A., and Ober, W. B. 1964. Fertility Sterility 15, 143.
1115. Maqueo, M., Perez-Vega, E., Goldzieher, J. W., Martinez-Manautou, J., and Rudel, H. 1963. Am. J. Obstet. Gynecol. 85, 427.
1116. Martinez-Manautou, J. M., Maqueo, M., Gilbert, R. A., and Goldzieher, J. W. 1962. Fertility Sterility 13, 169.
1117. Andreoli, C. 1962. Recenti Progr. Med. 32, 167.
1118. Durham, W. C. 1961. Fertility Sterility 12, 45.
1119. diPaola, G. 1963. Am. J. Obstet. Gynecol. 85, 421.
1120. D'Incerti-Bonini, L., and Pagani, C. 1961. Ann. Ostet. Ginecol. 83, 211.
1121. Greenblatt, R. B. 1958. Am. J. Obstet. Gynecol. 76, 626.
1122. Aydar, C. K., and Greenblatt, R. B. 1961. Acta Endocrinol. 38, 419.
1123. Greenblatt, R. B., and Rose, F. D. 1962. Obstet. Gynecol. 19, 730.
1124. Bishop, P. M. F., Borell, U., Diczfalusy, E., and Tillinger, K. G. 1962. Acta Endocrinol. 40, 203.
1125. Backer, M. H., Jr. 1962. Obstet. Gynecol. 15, 724.
1126. Venning, G. R. 1961. Brit. Med. J. II, 899.
1127. Garcia, C.-R., and Pincus, G. 1964. Intern. J. Fertility 9, 95.
1128. Rice-Wray, E., Goldzieher, J. W., and Aranda-Rosell, A. 1963. Fertility Sterility 14, 402.
1129. Cook, H. H., Gamble, C. J., and Satterthwaite, A. P. 1961. Am. J. Obstet. Gynecol. 82, 437.
1130. Tyler, E. T. 1961. J. Am. Med. Assoc. 175, 225.
1131. Morris, A. J., Jr. 1961. Am. J. Obstet. Gynecol. 82, 428.
1132. Mears, E. 1961. Brit. Med. J. II, 1179.
1133. Satterthwaite, A. P., and Gamble, C. J. 1962. J. Am. Med. Women's Assoc. 17, 797.

1134. Andrews, W. C., and Andrews, M. C. 1962. *Southern Med. J.* **55,** 454.

1135. Pullen, D. 1962. *Brit. Med. J.* **II,** 1016.

1136. Binks, R., Cambourn, P., and Papworth, R. A. 1962. *Med. J. Australia* I, 716.

1137. Gasset, J., and Gauthier, R. 1962. *Presse Med.* **70,** 9.

1138. Townsend, C. E. 1963. *Am. J. Obstet. Gynecol.* **87,** 130.

1139. Kitagawa, K., Ijiri, J., and Matsumiya, K. 1963. *Matsushita Bull. Human Sci.* **4,** 143.

1140. Wiseman, A. 1963. *Brit. Med. J.* **II,** 55.

1141. Shah, P. N. 1963. *J. Obstet. Gynecol. India* **13,** 14.

1142. Mears, E. 1963. *Family Planning* **12,** 61.

1143. Jackson, M. C. N. 1963. *J. Reprod. Fertility* **6,** 153.

1144. Rabbe, A., and Sorensen, H. B. 1964. *Ugeskrift Laeger* **126,** 100.

1145. Flowers, C. E., Jr. 1964. *J. Am. Med. Assoc.* **188,** 1115.

1146. Pincus, G. 1964. *Advan. Chem. Ser.* **49,** 177.

1147. Menon, K. 1964. *Proc. 7th Conf. Intern. Planned Parenthood Federation* p. 355.

1148. Chinnatamby, S. 1964. *Proc. 7th Intern. Conf. Planned Parenthood Federation* p. 319.

1149. Anderton, E. 1964. *Proc. 7th Intern. Conf. Planned Parenthood Federation* p. 389.

1150. Frank, R. 1964. *Proc. 7th Intern. Conf. Planned Parenthood Federation* p. 323.

1151. Peeters, F., van Roy, M., and Oeyen, H. 1960. *Geburtsh. Frauenheilk.* **20,** 1306.

1152. Mears, E., and Grant, E. C. G. 1962. *Brit. Med. J.* **II,** 75.

1153. Watts, G. F. 1962. *Am. J. Obstet. Gynecol.* **83,** 1132.

1154. Goldzieher, J. W., Moses, L. E., and Ellis, L. T. 1962. *J. Am. Med. Assoc.* **180,** 359.

1155. Bowman, R. 1962. *Med. J. Australia* I, 715.

1156. Mears, E. 1962. *J. Reprod. Fertility* **4,** 229.

1157. Bockner, V. 1963. *Med. J. Australia* I, 809.

1158. Swartz, D. P., Walters, J. H., Plunkett, E. R., and Kinch, R. A. H. 1963. *Fertility Sterility* **14,** 320.

1159. Ringrose, C. A. D. 1963. *Can. Med. Assoc. J.* **89,** 246.

1160. Symposium on Provest. 1963. *Intern. J. Fertility* p. 589 *et seq.*

1161. Andrews, W. C., and Andrews, M. C. 1964. *Fertility Sterility* **15,** 75.

1162. Kirchoff, H., and Haller, J. 1964. *Med. Klin. (Munich)* **59,** 681.

1163. Dukes, M. N. G., Kopera, H., and Ijzerman, G. L. 1964. *Proc. 7th Intern. Conf. Planned Parenthood Federation* p. 336.

1164. Swaab, L. I. 1964. *Prco. 7th Intern. Conf. Planned Parenthood Federation* p. 369.

1165. Garcia, C.-R., and Pincus, G. 1964. *Clin. Obstet. Gynecol.* **7,** 844.

1166. Pincus, G., Garcia, C.-R., Rocamora, H., and Curet, J. 1965. Unpublished data.

1167. Chinnatamby, S. 1964. Unpublished data.
1168. Venning, G. R. 1962. *Proc. Roy. Soc. Med.* **55**, 863.
1169. Holmes, R. L., and Mandl, A. M. 1962. *Lancet* **i,** 1174.
1170. Brown, J. B., Fotherby, K., and Loraine, J. A. 1962. *J. Endocrinol.* **25,** 331.
1171. Loraine, J. A., Bell, E. T., Harkness, R. A., Mears, E., and Jackson, M. C. N. 1963. *Lancet* **II,** 902.
1172. Bucholz, R., Nocke, L., and Nocke, W. 1962. *Geburtsh. Frauenheilk.* **22,** 923.
1173. Bucholz, R., Nocke, L., and Nocke, W. 1964. *Intern. J. Fertility* **9,** 231.
1174. Martin, L., and Cunningham, K. 1961. In "Human Pituitary Gonadotropins" (A. Albert, ed.), p. 226. C. C Thomas, Springfield, Illinois.
1175. Stevens, V. C., and Vorys, N. 1965. *Symp. on Recent Advan. Ovarian and Synthetic Steroids, Sydney, Australia.* In press.
1176. Szontagh, F. E., and Sas, M. 1962. *Gynaecologia* **154,** 81.
1177. Szontagh, F., Sas, M., Traub, A., Kovacs, L., Bardoczy, A., and Szereday, Z. 1963. *Orv. Hetilap* **104,** 1302.
1178. Lunenfeld, B., Sulimovici, S., and Raban, E. 1963. *J. Clin. Endocrinol. Metab.* **23,** 391.
1179. Diczfalusy, E. 1962. *Recent Progr. Hormone Res.* **18,** 381.
1180. Diczfalusy, E. 1965. *Symp. on Antifertility Agents.* In press.
1181. Arguelles, A. E., Saborida, C. M., and Chekherdemian, M. 1964. *Intern. J. Fertility* **9,** 217.
1182. Okada, H., Amatsu, M., Ishehara, S., and Tokuda, G. 1964. *Acta Endocrinol.* **46,** 31.
1183. Pincus, G. 1965. *Symp. on Antifertility Agents.* In press.
1184. Matsumoto, S., Ito, T., and Inone, S. 1960. *Geburtsh. Frauenheilk.* **20,** 250.
1185. Pincus, G. 1965. *Symp. on Recent Advan. Ovarian and Synthetic Steroids, Sydney, Australia.* In press.
1186. Eik-Nes, K. B. 1964. *Physiol. Revs.* **44,** 609.
1187. Siegel, I. 1963. *Obstet. Gynecol.* **21,** 666.
1188. Gold, J. J., Smith, L., Scommegna, A., and Borushek, S. 1963. *Intern. J. Fertility* **8,** 725.
1189. Fuchs, F., Johnsen, S. G., and Møeller, K. J. A. 1964. *Intern. J. Fertility* **9,** 147.
1190. Brown, P. S., Crooks, J., Klopper, A. I., Thorburn, A. R., and Tulloch, M. I. 1963. *Brit. Med. J.* **II,** 1630.
1191. Bell, E. T., Brown, J. B., Fotherby, K., Loraine, J. A., and Robson, J. S. 1962. *J. Endocrinol.* **25,** 221.
1192. Mears, E. 1962. *Lancet* **ii,** 614.
1193. Parkes, A. S. 1964. *Proc. 7th Intern. Conf. Planned Parenthood Federation* p. 493.

CHAPTER 12

Some Biological Properties of Ovulation Inhibitors in Human Subjects

The synthetic steroidal ovulation inhibitors are, as we have indicated previously, replicates of endogenous ovarian hormones. It is to be expected therefore that they will exhibit biological activities characteristic of these ovarian hormones. Since both estrogenic and progestational components are present in practically all of the ovulation-inhibiting preparations, target tissues for both progestin and estrogen will be affected depending on such factors as: (a) dosage, (b) estrogen-progestin interactions, (c) secondary effects from primary targets, (d) individual response thresholds, and (e) the degree of inhibition of endogenous ovarian hormone secretion. That each of these factors plays a role in the exhibition of the effects of progestin-estrogen combinations is exemplified by: (a) a dose-proportional incidence of breakthrough bleeding at doses which are completely effective contraceptively [1091 (Ch. 11)], (b) a degree of control of menstrual frequency and flow depending upon the estrogen used and the amount present in the given preparation [1083 (Ch. 11)], (c) the degree of protein binding of other hormones resulting from changes in blood concentration of specific hormone-labile binding proteins (1194), (d) the more than usual occurrence of breakthrough bleeding in some women, probably reflective of rather high dose requirements for the sustainment of endometrial vasculature (*1195*), (e) the reduction in pregnanediol output which varies from woman to woman [*926* (Ch. 9)], suggestive of ovarian thresholds to a suppressive action on endogenous progesterone production, or (f) the reduction in endogenous estrogen output [*1005* (Ch. 10), *1196*) which may compensate functionally for the estrogen added in the preparation used. Because of variations in the chemical configurations of the synthetic steroids used, one might perhaps find unusual effects never exhibited by the endogenous hormonal steroids. Actually, with perhaps one or two not adequately substantiated exceptions, no significant qualitative differences in effect have been reported, but quantitative variations are indeed indicated.

When we consider the multivarious activities of the ovarian hormones as primary or secondary regulators of numerous organ, tissue, and cellular processes (*1197*), it is not surprising to find an increasingly large literature on the physiological actions of the synthetic oral contraceptives. We shall attempt to present here primarily those which fairly regularly characterize their use in normal subjects. Since a completely normal woman is (fortunately!) primarily a statistic, some description of effects in abnormal states will be made, but primarily as these are relevant to an understanding of the physiological effects of the estrogen-progestin preparations. These effects may be analyzed as those involving (a) organs and functions primarily concerned with reproductive processes, (b) other endocrine glands and functions, and (c) other somatic tissues and metabolic activities.

Functions Associated with Reproductive Organs and Processes

OVARIES

We have described the effects of ovulation inhibitors on ovarian function in Chapter 11. The indicated lack of effect of Enovid on primary follicles [Table 42 and *1101* (Ch. 11)] has been reported for 17-methyl-19-nortestosterone (*1198*) and lynestrenol (*1199*). In ovaries from patients taking the last two substances, Ferin and his

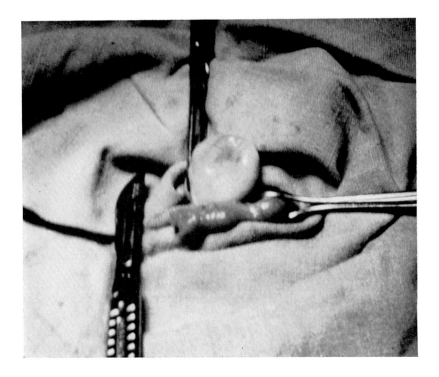

FIG. 20A. Inactive appearance of the ovary on the 29th day of a cycle in which Enovid (5 mg) was taken from day 5 to 25, and had been used for 64 consecutive cycles.

collaborators report a hemorrhagic thecal congestion not seen in ovaries similarly prevented from ovulation by the administration of stilbestrol (*1200*). The decrease in urinary estrogen excretion observed in women taking steroid preparations is not simply the result of the prevention of corpus luteum formation since several women with gonadal dysgenesis demonstrated a similar decrease during medication with medroxyprogesterone (*1201*). Also, Taymor

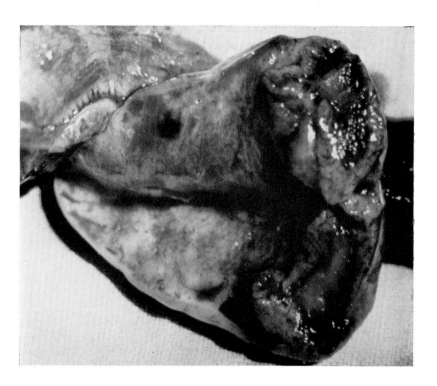

Fig. 20B. Well-developed corpus luteum in a patient examined 5½ weeks after cessation of Enovid medication; she had been taking Enovid for 5 years previous to cessation.

(*1202*) has demonstrated that the urinary output of both total gonadotropin and of LH by patients taking norethindrone acetate is decreased before midcycle. This is paralleled by quite low pregnanediol outputs, suggesting that maintenance of steroidogenesis in the nonluteal tissue is had by gestagen-labile gonadotropic factors. Here again a direct effect on ovarian secretions is not altogether excluded since breakthrough ovulation at these suppressive doses has been claimed (*1203*).

On the other hand, the dithiocarbamoylhydrazine which effectively reduces gonadotropin excretion in postmenopausal women [1191 (Ch. 11)] has no such effect in pregnant mares (1204) or in cycling women (1205). Yet when it is administered to the latter before ovulation, urinary estrogen, pregnanediol, and pregnanetriol excretion is decreased and no such decrease is seen during postovulatory administration [as with post-ovulatory Enovid administration [1083 (Ch. 11)]. It is thus possible that ovarian steroidogenesis in tissues other than the corpus luteum is labile to some ovulation inhibitors but not to others. Once a functional corpus luteum is established, inhibition of its steroid-secreting capacity is not easily accomplished. This suggests that luteal steroid production may not be regulated by LH nor even by FSH but by a luteotropic hormone (i.e., LTH). This is certainly true in the rat where LTH is prolactin [36 (Ch. 2)], but human LTH is certainly not prolactin and its reality yet remains to be demonstrated.

Although much remains to be determined concerning the exact results of the use of ovulation inhibitors upon various ovarian tissues and functions, all observers are agreed that cessation of use is followed by prompt recovery of normal function. Most obvious is the prompt occurrence of conception in users of various oral contraceptives following discontinuance of use [1090, 1091, 1188 (Ch. 11); 1206]. Indeed, Goldzieher et al. (1207) find a doubling of the expected conception rate during the first month after discontinuance of use of a norethindrone-estrogen combination. In Fig. 20 we present photographs taken at laparotomy of two human ovaries, the first (A) showing the small corpus-luteum-free ovary of a woman on Enovid therapy for several years; the second (B) showing the large corpus luteum established at 5½ weeks after withdrawal from Enovid therapy after similar long-term use. In addition to the prompt return of ovulation and luteal function, a normal cyclical pattern of urinary steroid excretion is established, and this has been seen in users of 19-norsteroid and acetoxyprogesterone derivatives (1208).

UTERUS

Since the uterus is a primary target organ for estrogens and progestins, it is in this organ that we should and do observe characteristic effects of the contraceptive preparations. Those most completely described are (a) endometrial biopsies taken at various times during each treatment cycle and (b) variations in menstrual phenomena such as cycle lengths, nature, and duration of the menstrual flow and various menstrual irregularities.

A typical sequence of histological change occurs during any given day 5 through 24 cycle of use of estrogen-progestin combinations [*1083, 1119* (Ch. 11)]. Depending somewhat on dosage and the preparations used, one observes on the first day or two a continuation of the proliferative type of endometrium, then a rapid development of a typical secretory phase culminating in a few days into the type of endometrium seen at days 19 to 20 of the typical menstrual cycle. There then follows a period during which the endometrial glands undergo a greater or lesser degree of involution *pari passu* with the development of varying degrees of stromal edema, often culminating in a predecidual or pseudodecidual condition. Upon withdrawal of the medication, bleeding occurs from this characteristic "hormonal" endometrium. This sequence of changes is illustrated in Fig. 21.

In Table 43 we present the categorization of the endometrial biopsies taken from subjects in San Juan before undertaking the use of Enovid, following withdrawal from use after one or more years and during use for various numbers of lunar years. Specimens were taken as the patients appeared for examination and are at random in terms of the specific day of the menstrual cycle. These biopsies were examined by a cytologist who had no knowledge of the time of cycle, the use or nonuse of medication. The first three categories are self-explanatory; that designated "hormonal effect" includes specimens showing the typical stromal edema accompanied by varying degrees of glandular involution described above; "dysplasias" are primarily cystic and adenomatous hyperplasias with a small proportion of anaplasias; endometritis is obvious and the last category includes a few mildly atypical conditions. The most notable features of the data of this table are: (a) the reduced frequency of occurrence of typical proliferative and secretory endometria in Enovid users, (b) the consistent high proportion of "hormonal effect" specimens in Enovid users, (c) the consistent reduced frequency of dysplasia and endometritis in Enovid users,

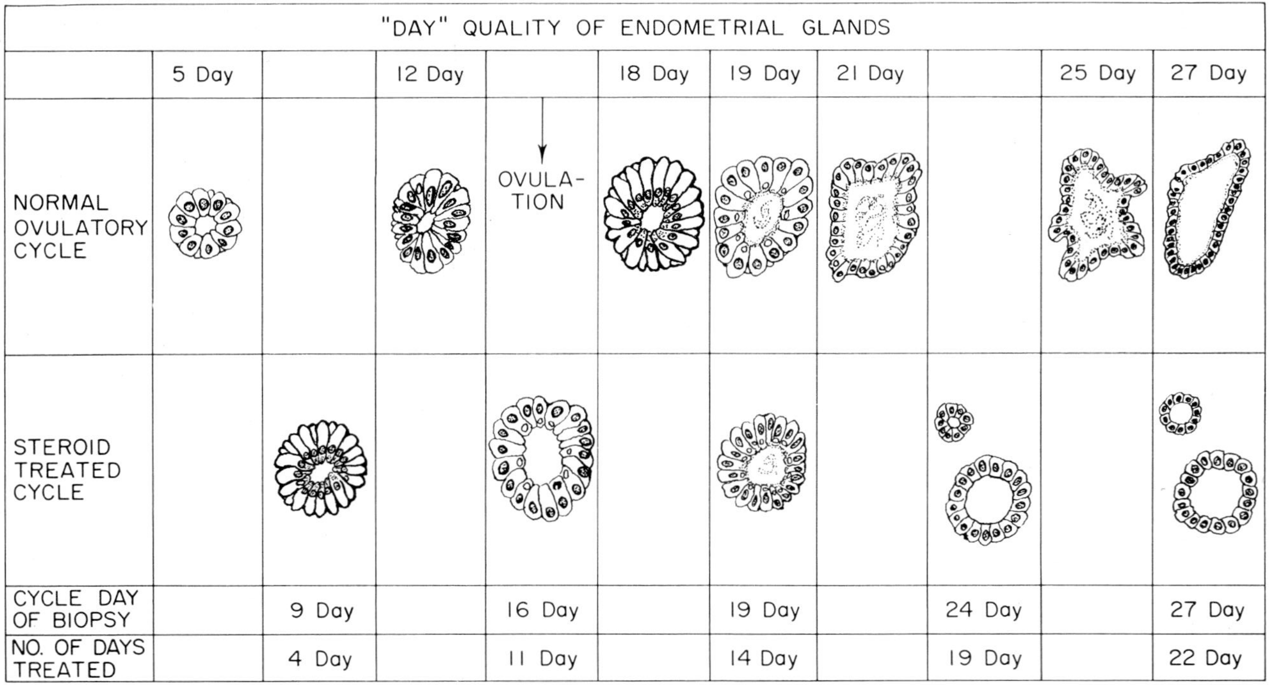

"DAY" QUALITY OF ENDOMETRIAL GLANDS

	5 Day		12 Day	OVULA-TION	18 Day	19 Day	21 Day	25 Day	27 Day
NORMAL OVULATORY CYCLE									
STEROID TREATED CYCLE									
CYCLE DAY OF BIOPSY		9 Day		16 Day		19 Day		24 Day	27 Day
NO. OF DAYS TREATED		4 Day		11 Day		14 Day		19 Day	22 Day

Fig. 21. Appearance of endometrial glands in normal and in Enovid-treated cycles.

and (d) the return to the premedication pattern in the subjects discontinuing use. The occurrence in the latter of "hormonal effect" specimens is somewhat above the premedication frequency and may represent a carry-over of a degree of glandular regression noted by other observers in specimens from women discontinuing use of other progestin-estrogen combinations (*1207, 1209*). The

TABLE 43

ENDOMETRIAL BIOPSIES OF ENOVID USERS (SAN JUAN)

		% with						
Type of subject	No.	Prolif- erative	Secre- tory	Men- strual	Hor- monal effect	Dys- plasia	Endo- metritis	Miscel- laneous
Premedication	231	44	25	6	10	5	9	2
Enovid, 1 yr	113	13	7	7	70	2	1	—
Enovid, 2 yr	145	4	8	7	79	1	2	—
Enovid, 3 yr	131	10	6	9	73	2	1	—
Enovid, 4 yr	96	10	5	9	72	1	1	—
Enovid, 5–8 yr	94	9	13	3	69	—	4	2
Withdrawn	64	33	28	5	22	2	6	5

rapid return to usual endometrial sequences is seen in electron microscopic patterns observed in endometria of women discontinuing use of Enovid and Norlutate (*1210*). The remarkable consistency of the biopsy pattern seen year after year in Enovid users is indicative of the constancy of the degree of hormonal stimulation consequent on the use of a standard estrogen-progestin combination.

In a comparative study of biopsies taken from subjects taking either norethynodrel, norethindrone, or chlormadinone as the gestagen, Maqueo *et al.* (*1115*) find practically superimposable patterns of development during medication in measures of glandular tortuosity, secretory changes, stromal edema, and predecidual changes (*1211*). This is illustrated in Fig. 22 where their estimate of degree of change is based on an arbitrary scale for each condition varying from 0 to 4. Again, the notable similarity of pattern by these measures in users of preparations containing three chemically

A

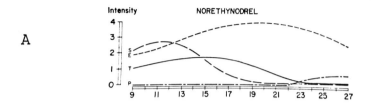

B

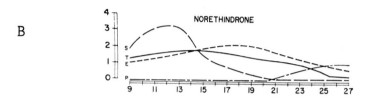

C

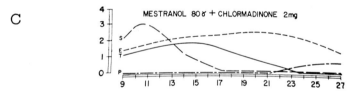

Fɪɢ. 22. Variations in glandular tortuosity (T), secretory changes (S), stromal edema (E), and pseudodecidual changes (P) during cycles of use of Enovid (10 mg) (A); Orthonovum (10 mg) (B); and Lutoral (2 mg) (C).

dissimilar gestagens suggests the importance to the endometrium of a constant progestin-estrogen hormonal milieu.

This regularly maintained milieu is also responsible for a significant regularization of menstrual phenomena. We early noticed that the variability in menstrual cycle lengths characteristic of a group of presumably normal, healthy women is very much reduced in users of Enovid, 10 mg (1212). The standard deviation of mean cycle lengths was approximately 60% of that observed in Haman's (*1213*) data for 2410 cycles of 150 normal subjects. This reduced variability was due to a reduced frequency of both short (7–25 days) and long (29–48 days) cycles. A similar relative infrequency

TABLE 44

MEAN CYCLE LENGTHS IN ENOVID USERS

Lunar years of use	Mean cycle lengths in days at		
	2.5 mg/day	5 mg/day	10 mg/day
1	25.7 ± 0.10[a]	25.8 ± 0.07[a]	26.6 ± 0.09[a]
2	26.1 ± 0.07	26.0 ± 0.07	26.7 ± 0.09
3	26.2 ± 0.07	26.1 ± 0.07	26.4 ± 0.24
4	26.2 ± 0.09	26.4 ± 0.06	28.7 ± 0.68
5	26.2 ± 0.26	26.4 ± 0.10	27.3 ± 0.87
6	27.2 ± 0.32	26.4 ± 0.11	—
7	27.4 ± 0.28	26.5 ± 0.17	—
8	26.4 ± 0.34	26.1 ± 0.24	—

[a] ± standard error.

of short and long cycle lengths has been reported for over 6000 cycles of use of Orthonovum, 10 mg [*1154* (Ch. 11)]. The remarkable constancy of mean menstrual cycle lengths from year to year in long-term users is illustrated in Table 44 which demonstrates a recurring 26- to 27-day mean; a somewhat shorter mean duration

TABLE 45

MEAN CYCLE LENGTHS (DAYS) IN 200 WOMEN USING
VAGINAL CONTRACEPTIVES AND 200 WOMEN USING ENOVID (5 MG)

Contraceptive	Cycle 1	Cycle 3	Cycle 5
Vaginal	31.5	30.0	31.6
Enovid	26.8	25.8	26.5

in the first year of use of 2.5 and 5 mg dosages is presumably reflective of a certain amount of tablet-missing with consequent withdrawal flow and a shortened cycle.

We have recently compared menstrual cycle phenomena in 200 women taking Enovid (5 mg) and 200 using a vaginal contraceptive. The assignment to Enovid or the vaginal contraceptive was randomized and in the same Puerto Rican population. In Table 45 we list the mean cycle lengths observed in the first, third, and fifth cycles of use. It is obvious that Enovid in these cycles imposes a characteristic cycle shorter than that seen in nonusers in which a mean latent period to flow of 1.8 to 2.8 days follows the last day (i.e., 24) of use. When we determined the degree of irregularity

TABLE 46

DEGREE OF MENSTRUAL REGULARITY IN FIRST FIVE CYCLES OF
CONTRACEPTIVE USE

(subjects as in Table 45)

Contraceptive	% with differences of 5 days or less between maximal and minimal cycle lengths	% with differences of more than 5 days between maximal and minimal cycle lengths	% with amenorrhea in one cycle
Vaginal	36.1	50.2	13.7
Enovid	58.9	37.2	3.9

in length from cycle to cycle in these same women we have the data presented in Table 46, which shows that approximately 59% of the Enovid users have had cycles differing from each other by 5 days or less in length whereas 36% of the vaginal contraceptive users showed this degree of regularity. Furthermore, the nonusers

TABLE 47

MEAN DURATION (IN DAYS) OF MENSTRUATION IN CONTRACEPTIVE USERS

(subjects as in Table 45)

Contraceptive	Cycle 1	Cycle 2	Cycle 5
Vaginal	4.3	4.1	3.9
Enovid	3.9	3.9	3.7

of Enovid had a much higher frequency of occurrence of amenorrheic cycles. By ordinary standards then 63.9% of the vaginal contraceptive users exhibited menstrual irregularity over a 5-cycle period whereas 41.1% of the Enovid users were irregular. When we consider that these first 5 cycles represent those in which pill forgetting and/or adjustment to the medication occurs, it is clear that the irregularities will be even less manifest in longer term use. Not only is menstrual cycle length fairly strictly regulated, but also the duration and quality of the menstrual flow. Among oral contraceptive users there is exhibited a somewhat shortened mean

TABLE 48

MEAN DURATION OF MENSTRUATION (IN DAYS) IN USERS OF
ENOVID, 2.5 MG; ORTHONOVUM, 2 MG; OVULEN, 1 MG

Cycle No.	No. of subjects	Enovid	No. of subjects	Orthonovum	No. of subjects	Ovulen
1	155	4.4	147	4.2	124	4.2
4	167	4.0	160	3.6	124	3.6
13	115	3.9	117	3.3	92	3.8
26	53	3.2	59	3.3	24	2.8

duration of menstruation (Table 47). The data of a comparative study of users of three 19-norsteroid-estrogen combinations demonstrate a tendency to shortening of mean durations of menstruation in the course of 2 years of use (Table 48). Along with the decrease in average duration there is also a decrease in the amount of the

TABLE 49

PERCENTAGE OF SUBJECTS CLAIMING LIGHTER OR
HEAVIER MENSTRUAL FLOW

(subjects as in Table 45)

	Cycle 1		Cycle 3		Cycle 5	
Contraceptive	Heavier	Lighter	Heavier	Lighter	Heavier	Lighter
Vaginal	8.0	9.6	6.4	2.5	3.2	4.3
Enovid	9.8	13.4	8.6	10.6	4.1	10.7

menstrual discharge. This is illustrated in Table 49 which summarizes the claimed change in amount of menstrual flow in users of a vaginal or of an oral contraceptive. It demonstrates that the claimed occurrence of heavier flow drops to low levels from the first to the fifth cycle of use in both groups, but the observation of lighter flows in Enovid users is higher than and more sustained than in vaginal contraceptive users. In the comparative study described in Table 48 14 to 18% of users observed lighter flows in the course of a year [1146 (Ch. 11)], and Mears [1107 (Ch. 11)] reports reduction in menstrual flow in 20 to 85% of users of six progestin-estrogen combinations varying somewhat from preparation and with dosage and duration of use. The use of these preparations in the control of hypermenorrhea (1214–1216) has now become a well-established clinical practice and has often obviated the need for hysterectomy (1217). With Ovulen, the control may be exercised either by the usual day 5 to 25 regimen or with post-ovulatory administration from day 15 to 25 (1218). This indicates that control of flow involves a direct action on the endometrium and not via pituitary inhibition. Klopper (1219) finds that on discontinuance of use the premedication pattern of dysfunctional flow tends to return.

Although the data on control by estrogen-progestin combinations of menstrual cyclicity and flow are unequivocal, an apparent exception is observed in the occurrence of menstrual spotting or bleeding during the period of use. This has been denominated breakthrough bleeding (BTB). The proportion of cycles in which BTB occurred in subjects taking Enovid is shown in Table 50.

TABLE 50

PERCENTAGE OF CYCLES SHOWING SPOTTING OR BLEEDING (BTB)
DURING ENOVID ADMINISTRATION

Cycle No.	No. cycles	2.5 mg % with BTB	No. cycles	5 mg % with BTB	No. cycles	10 mg % with BTB
1	223	28.3	766	13.4	1065	6.4
2	197	23.4	749	11.9	901	4.2
10–19	618	13.1	5503	4.7	2903	2.2
30–39	294	11.2	2729	3.8	167	3.0
50–59	106	4.7	674	4.0	—	—

This demonstrates (a) a maximal occurrence of BTB in the first cycle of use in all three groups, (b) a decline to low levels thereafter, and (c) a rate of occurrence roughly inversely proportional to the dose. This first cycle maximum and later decline has been seen by several observers using a number of estrogen-progestin mixtures [e.g., *1107* (Ch. 11), *1220*]. There appears to be some variation with the particular gestagenic component; thus in Mexico, Rice-Wray (*1220*) finds the percentages of first cycle BTB's as follows: Lutoral (2 mg), 15.7; Enovid (5 mg), 9.5; Lyndiol (5 mg), 5.2; Orthonovum (5 mg), 3.2. We have some data suggesting that BTB may be associated with missing of pill taking. This is presented in Table 51 where it is seen that in the 219 cycles in which no missing of tablet taking was claimed only one short cycle was reported, whereas when 1 to 5 tablets were missed two thirds of the cycles were shortened. It is conceivable, therefore, that first cycle BTB is in some measure associated with getting used to daily pill taking. Actually, when the percentage of BTB falls below 10% a better than normal control of cycle length is suggested since

TABLE 51
PILL TAKING AND SHORT CYCLES (LESS THAN 24 DAYS) IN OVULEN USERS

No. of pills missed	No. of cycles	% of total cycles	No. of short cycles	% of short cycles
0	219	93	1	0.5
1–5	14	6	4	67
6–19	3	1	3	100

Haman's data (*1213*) reveal that 10% of "normal" cycles are less than 24 days in length (cf. *1221*). However, the differences in BTB seen from preparation to preparation do not appear to be due to chance forgettings. As Table 50 demonstrates, a dosage-response relationship is indicated and this has not been established for other preparations so that this may be a matter merely of endometrium-maintaining potency of the gestagen, or, as we have previously indicated, a function of the dosage and nature of the estrogenic component. The ratio of progestin to estrogen also plays a role as Hisaw and Hisaw (*1222*) have demonstrated in castrated monkeys where endometria sustained by the administration of 10 μg per day of estradiol will exhibit BTB when progesterone is administered in daily doses of 0.06 to 0.5 mg, but will not exhibit BTB when the daily progesterone dose is raised to 0.7 mg.

A notable effect on endometrial pathology is seen in the action of synthetic gestagen-estrogen combinations upon endometriosis.

Following the observation that pregnancy improves this condition, Kistner (*1223, 1224*) employed continuous administration of large doses and several preparations (*1225*) for many months with significant regression of endometriosis. These observations have been repeated by a number of investigators, principally with Enovid (*1226–1228*), but also with other preparations (*1229*) including the use of a gestagen alone (*1230*). The remarkable reduction in pain, the clearing up of lesions in distant sites (*1231, 1232*), and the general symptom relief has led to the use of brief, small-dose administration for the diagnosis of endometriosis (*1233*). Conservative surgery as a follow-up to long-term gestagen-estrogen administration may lead to a permanent cure since on cessation of hormone administration, recurrence may occur (*1234*) but in a number of cases pregnancies have been established where previously there seemed no possibility of them in the presence of the active disease.

That estrogen-progestin mixtures administered during the menstrual cycle affect pain and distress associated with menstruation has been known for some time. Enovid was originally reported to decrease dysmenorrhea (*1235*) and premenstrual tension (*1236*) in women habitually afflicted with these conditions. In our con-

TABLE 52

CHANGES IN OCCURRENCE OF DYSMENORRHEA
DURING USE OF CONTRACEPTIVES

(subjects as in Table 45)

	% with preRx pain reporting none			% with no preRx pain reporting some		
Contraceptive	Cycle 1	Cycle 3	Cycle 5	Cycle 1	Cycle 3	Cycle 5
Vaginal	48	30	54	10	10	8
Enovid	66	77	84	4.5	9.0	7.1

trolled series of vaginal contraceptive and Enovid users the women with dysmenorrhea previous to use reported lack of pain in 30 to 54% of cycles with vaginal contraceptives but in 66 to 84% of cycles with Enovid (Table 52). Appearance of dysmenorrhea in women not reporting its premedication occurrence was somewhat but not significantly less in Enovid users. The proportion of women reporting the occurrence of dysmenorrhea at least once in a year differs markedly in the two areas where our study projects have been conducted. This is indicated by the data of Table 53 where 24% of Haitian women report dysmenorrhea in a premedication year in contrast to 52% of Puerto Rican women. Both groups have lower incidence while using Enovid. Wiseman (*1237*) finds that 54% of patients attending her clinic in Slough report dysmenorrhea, but in users of Ovulen this drops to 16% with a mild discomfort after three cycles.

In studies of patients with functional dysmenorrhea Bishop and Cabral de Almeida (*1238*) found relief of dysmenorrhea in 65 of 91 cycles in which norethisterone was administered on days 5 to 25, but they claimed no relief occurred if administration was initiated

TABLE 53
DYSMENORRHEA

Clinic location	Treatment	No. of subjects	% with dysmenorrhea
San Juan	Premedication *Enovid*	230	52 ± 3.3[a]
	1st yr	127	35 ± 4.3
	2nd yr	132	48 ± 4.4
	3rd yr	129	44 ± 4.4
	4th yr	83	46 ± 5.5
	5–7th yr	56	46 ± 6.7
	Withdrawn	58	47 ± 6.6
Haiti	Premedication *Enovid*	29	24 ± 8.1
	1st yr	43	12 ± 5.0
	2nd yr	36	8 ± 4.6
	3rd yr	37	19 ± 6.5

[a] ± standard error.

after day 6. The relief was therefore ascribed to a central ovulation-inhibiting effect. In contrast, Bertrand et al. (*1239*) find that norethynodrel taken after ovulation is quite effective in the relief of congestive dysmenorrhea. In a later paper, Bishop (*1240*) finds that 6-dehydroretroprogesterone (Duphaston) is quite effective in producing painless uterine bleeding, although it fails to suppress

TABLE 54

THE OCCURRENCE OF ENDOMETRIAL DYSPLASIAS AND OF ENDOMETRITIS

Clinic location	Type of subject	Number examined	% with dysplasias	Endometritis
San Juan	Premedication	231	5.1 ± 1.45^b	9.4 ± 1.92^b
	Enovid users	579	$\underline{1.5^a} \pm 0.51$	$\underline{1.3} \pm 0.47$
	Postmedication	64	2.2 ± 1.85	6.0 ± 2.99
Haiti	Premedication	872	9.1 ± 0.97	9.8 ± 1.01
	Enovid users	336	$\underline{3.8} \pm 1.04$	$\underline{3.6} \pm 1.02$
	Vaginal contraceptive users	131	$\underline{6.4} \pm 2.14$	$\underline{4.1} \pm 1.74$

[a] Underlined values differ significantly from premedication values.
[b] $\pm$ standard error.

ovulation. He contrasts this with similar effects of norethindrone at ovulation-suppressing doses and concludes that two mechanisms may operate—one as a result of induced anovulation, the other directly on the uterus. Although day 5 to 25 administration of other gestagens or progestin-estrogen mixtures have also led to symptom-free cycles (*1241*), a detailed analysis of the mechanism of their action remains to be determined.

The "normalization" of uterine function indicated by the menstrual regularities described above is also accompanied by a tendency to bring back to normal uteri of abnormal size or in abnormal states. We have already commented on the reduction in

TABLE 55

PALPABLE SURFACE OF THE FUNDUS

Treatment	Dose (mg)	No. of subjects	% Hypoplastic	Normal	Hyper- plastic	Ill- defined
Premedication	—	428	3 ± 0.8^a	43 ± 2.4^a	48 ± 2.4	5 ± 1.0^a
Enovid	10	197	4 ± 1.4	82 ± 2.7	11 ± 2.2	4 ± 1.4
Enovid	5	1127	3 ± 0.5	81 ± 1.2	12 ± 3.1	4 ± 0.6
Enovid	2.5	357	3 ± 0.9	71 ± 2.4	22 ± 2.2	3 ± 0.9
Ovulen	1–2	150	2 ± 1.2	87 ± 2.8	9 ± 2.3	1 ± 0.8
Withdrawn	—	161	3 ± 1.3	72 ± 3.5	22 ± 3.3	3 ± 1.3

[a] $\pm$ standard error.

occurrence of dysplasias and endometritis in Enovid users in San Juan (Table 43). This is seen also in Haiti where cystic and adenomatous endometrial hyperplasia is more frequent than in Puerto Rico (Table 54). The reduction over premedication incidence is clear and Enovid users tend to have lower incidences than users of vaginal contraceptives. Rather high premedication incidence of uterine hyperplasia observed at pelvic examination of volunteers in Puerto Rico is shown in the data of Table 55. A return to normal size is indicated in the users of Enovid and Ovulen.

CERVIX

Cervix consistency as determined by palpation at physical examination is classified in Table 56. There are no consistent changes observed in oral contraceptive users. The reduction in the proportion of firm cervices in Ovulen users is accompanied by an increase

TABLE 56
CERVIX CONSISTENCY ON PALPATION

		\% classified as			
Treatment	No.	Firm	Soft	Irregular	Rough	Smooth
---	---	---	---	---	---	---
Premedication	365	67 ± 2.5^a	5 ± 1.1^a	5 ± 1.1^a	12 ± 1.7^a	10 ± 1.6^a
Enovid, 10 mg	157	75 ± 3.5	9 ± 2.3	11 ± 2.5	$\underline{1 \pm 0.8^b}$	4 ± 1.6
Enovid, 5 mg	913	66 ± 1.6	$\underline{18 \pm 1.3}$	7 ± 0.8	$\underline{4 \pm 0.6}$	6 ± 0.8
Enovid, 2.5 mg	351	76 ± 2.3	$\underline{4 \pm 1.0}$	6 ± 1.3	$\underline{8 \pm 1.4}$	6 ± 1.3
Ovulen, 1–2 mg	68	$\underline{40 \pm 6.0}$	3 ± 2.1	4 ± 2.4	18 ± 4.7	$\underline{35 \pm 5.8}$
Withdrawn	137	$\underline{76 \pm 3.7}$	10 ± 2.6	3 ± 1.5	$\underline{3 \pm 1.5}$	8 ± 2.3

[a] $\pm$ standard error.
[b] Underlined values differ significantly from premedication values.

in the proportion classified as smooth. The significant increase in the "soft" category in Enovid (5 mg) users is not seen in the other two Enovid dosage groups. There does appear to be some tendency for a reduction in cervices classified as "rough" in Enovid users in subjects after discontinuing oral contraception.

The state of the cervical mucus in users of oral contraceptives has been described by Zanartu (*1242*) who finds that during medication "there was a rapid and progressive change toward progestational-like characteristics, which established themselves even before or at about midcycle." The midcycle peak of thread-ability is abolished, viscosity is increased, ferning is inhibited, and sperm penetration and motility decrease in Sims-Hühner tests performed at 2 to 12 hours after fertile coitus. The decreased penetrability to sperm of mucus from Enovid users was described by Guard (1243) using an improved method of determining rates of sperm movement. Since sperm normally penetrates to a greater or lesser extent into cervical mucus throughout the cycle (1244),

TABLE 57
CERVICAL EROSIONS

Treatment	Dosage (mg)	Number	% with erosions
Premedication	—	393	46 ± 2.5[a]
Enovid withdrawn	—	163	51 ± 3.9
Enovid	10	199	63[b] ± 3.4
Enovid	5	1081	65 ± 1.5
Enovid	2.5	375	71 ± 2.4
Ovulen premedication	—	64	69 ± 5.8
Ovulen	1–2	69	74 ± 5.3

[a] ± standard error.
[b] Underlined values differ significantly from premedication values.

a hypergestational effect is suggested by Zanartu's observations. The mechanisms involved in cervical mucus changes are not too clear. According to Beller and Vogler (1245) the natural estrogens decrease cervical mucus consistency, but progesterone has no direct effect and acts only as an estrogen antagonist. A careful study of local vs. systemic administration effects of various progestin-estrogen combinations would be quite worthwhile.

The cervices of users of Enovid when seen at pelvic examination may at times appear somewhat hyperemic. This suggests a stimulatory effect by the steroids. On the other hand, it may represent a mild inflammatory reaction to hormone-conditioned environment. In Puerto Rico and Haiti the high prevalence of cervical erosions has been recognized, and typical figures are presented in Table 57. It may be seen that 46% of the Enovid users examined before use had erosions. In examinations made during the use of Enovid, the occurrence increased to from 63 to 71%. This increase has been attributed to a softening of the cervices in Enovid users [*1129* (Ch. 11)]. It should be noted that though the occurrence in Ovulen users is high it is not significantly different from the frequency in premedication examinations; more recently we have found no significant change in postmedication erosion incidence in a large group of women seen at least once during a 2-year period of use. There may therefore be a difference in the action of these two preparations upon the cervix, or it may be that latterly the examining physicans have been more alert to detecting smaller erosions particularly.

In the course of our studies with volunteer subjects taking Enovid for contraception, we obtained routinely vaginal smears which were stained by the method of Papanicolaou. In examining the diagnoses for the several hundred smears we were surprised to find only one (or 0.2%) recorded as suspicious, i.e., Papanicolaou Grade III [*1091* (Ch. 11)], since Lee *et al.* (*1246*) had observed a prevalence figure of 4.4% for vaginal smears graded III (3.3%),

TABLE 58

THE PREVALENCE OF SUSPICIOUS PAPANICOLAOU SMEARS
IN VARIOUS EXPERIMENTAL STUDY AREAS IN SUBJECTS
PREVIOUS TO CONTRACEPTIVE USE

Area	Number of women	Suspicious smears per 1000 women
Rio Piedras, P.R.	1920	29.2
Humacao, P.R.	1527	30.8
Port-au-Prince	1091	29.3
Mexico City	297	3.0
San Antonio	289	10.3
Colombo	250	12.0

IV (0.5%), or V (0.6%) in Puerto Rican women. This finding suggested a possible suppressive action of the progestin-estrogen combination upon atypical cellular growth. Accordingly we embarked upon a larger scale survey to determine the suitability of our study population for a controlled incidence study. Papanicolaou smears from the vaginal pool and the surface of the cervix were obtained. In Table 58 we present the data on the prevalence of smears of Grade III or higher at six study clinics. It is clear that those in

Puerto Rico and Haiti have a much higher occurrence than those in Mexico, Texas, and Ceylon. Accordingly, we have concentrated our studies in the Caribbean centers. We have presented (*1247*) comparative incidence figures for five groups of subjects in these areas (Table 59). The new suspicious smears appearing are practically exclusively Grade III, and represent a cervical anaplastic cellular exfoliate. It is obvious that the users of the three contraceptive preparations have a much lower rate of occurrence of such anaplasia than the users of vaginal contraceptives or of intrauterine contraceptive devices. This may be due to the local irritation caused

TABLE 59

THE RATE OF DEVELOPMENT OF SUSPICIOUS PAPANICOLAOU SMEARS IN SUBJECTS WITH NEGATIVE SMEARS BEFORE THE USE OF VARIOUS CONTRACEPTIVES

Contraceptive used	Number of subjects	Number/1,000 with suspicious smears
Vaginal	208	72.1 ± 18.0^a
Enovid	580	$\underline{26.2^b} \pm 6.6$
Ovulen	188	$\underline{21.3} \pm 10.5$
Orthonovum	105	28.6 ± 16.4
Intrauterine devices	500	54.0 ± 10.0

[a] $\pm$ standard error.
[b] Underlined values differ significantly from those for vaginal contraceptives.

by the latter two methods, or it may indicate a preventive effect of the estrogen-progestin mixtures upon abnormal cellular growth in the cervix. Evidence for a preventive effect is seen in the data of Table 60, which lists the percentage of type III smears seen at various intervals after the entry of 651 subjects into the use of intrauterine devices (IUCD), of 515 into the use of vaginal contraceptives and of 769 into the use of Enovid (5 mg). In all three groups the proportion exhibiting type III smears increases with time, but from 11 to 15 months on it is minimal in the Enovid users. Patients entering the study with suspicious smears tend to continue to show such smears at a somewhat lower frequency in Enovid users (*1247*). The occurrence of cervical carcinoma as revealed by cervical biopsy is as yet quite low in our subjects, and the data to mid-1964 are presented in Table 61. The carcinomas listed as occurring "de novo" were observed after a year or longer in patients originally exhibiting negative smears. These may indeed have been false negatives since the smear is certainly not 100%

TABLE 60

RATE OF OCCURRENCE OF ANAPLASTIC SMEARS IN CONTRACEPTIVE USERS
WITH NEGATIVE SMEARS AT ENTRY

Cycles No.	I.U.C.D.		Intravaginal		Enovid (5 mg)	
	No. of subjects at start	% Positive	No. of subjects at start	% Positive	No. of subjects at start	% Positive
1–5	651	0.4	515	0.1	769	0.6
6–10	560	2.5	356	0.4	654	0.6
11–15	355	4.2	216	3.4	532	2.1
16–20	204	7.0	60	12.4	193	4.0
21–25	102	8.0	21	15.6	118	2.6

revelatory of the exact cervical tissue state. The suggestion of a prophylactic effect of estrogen-progestin mixtures upon abnormal tissue growth in the cervix obviously requires much further inquiry, and we are now engaged in a large-scale study in which

TABLE 61

SUMMARY OF THE OCCURRENCE OF CERVICAL BIOPSIES WITH CARCINOMA

Contraceptive used	Total number of biopsies	Number with carcinoma	% with carcinoma
Vaginal	41	4[a]	9.8
Coils	15	1[b]	6.7
Orals	185	8[c]	4.3
Controls	101	7	6.9

[a] 2 de novo.
[b] 1 de novo.
[c] 1 de novo.

assignment to an oral contraceptive is randomized against assignment to a vaginal spermicidal jelly or cream.

When we turn to the literature for guidance as to possible involvement of hormonal factors in cancer of the uterus and cervix, we are met with some agreements and some apparent bewildering contradictions [860 (Ch. 8)]. The premalignant lesions of the endometrium appear to be reflective of a hyperestrinism (1248). Moreover, a remarkable record of remissions in cases of advanced carcinoma of the endometrium with metastatic lesions treated with progesterone has been reported by Kelley and Baker (1250, 1251). A regressive effect of a depot progestin (Delalutin) in some endometrial carcinomas has been seen (1252). The oral gestagens, medroxyprogesterone and 17α-vinylestr-4-en-3-one-17-ol, have been therapeutically effective in a number of cases of adenocarcinomic and anaplastic endometrial hyperplasia; in the latter condition a prophylactic anticarcinogenic effect was suggested (1253, 1254). Neither lynestrenol alone nor lynestrenol in combination with an estrogen enhanced cancer induction or progression in rats and women (1255). Inhibition of mitoses in endometrial carcinoma has been observed following 2 weeks of administration of various gestagens (1249). No tumoricidal or growth-inhibiting effects have been seen in corpus sarcomas or mixed mesodermal tumors of the corpus (1256). In guinea pigs, estrogen-dependent uterine fibromas may be inhibited by androgen or progestin administration (1257), and in rabbits inhibition by synthetic progestin administration of carcinogen induction of endometrial carcinoma in estrogenized animals has been reported (1258). The suggestion is, therefore, of an anti-estrogenic action of gestagens in endometrial carcinoma; one would expect an increased rate of occurrence of endometrial carcinoma in women with a marked progesterone deficiency or excessive endogenous or exogenous estrogen, and this has indeed been claimed (1259, 1260).

Athough the occurrence after some years of fibromyomas in a number of women having endometrial hyperplasia has been attributed to the unopposed action of endogenous estrogen (1261), stilbestrol administration has led to no increases in fibromyoma size (1262). The observation of increase in myoma size in pregnancy seems to be paralleled by a stimulative effect of a progestin-estrogen combination on fibromyomata (1263). However, in our project patients we have not noted any stimulative effect on existing fibromyomata in long-term users of Enovid, Orthonovum, and Ovulen, and Wiseman (1237) found no significant changes in fibromyomata sizes in Ovulen users.

In the case of cancer of the cervix, indications of hormone involvement are more obscure. In mice with carcinogen placed in the cervix ovariectomy appears to promote the development of invasive tumors (*1264*), prolonged estrogen treatment of mice has led eventually to carcinoma induction [*860* (Ch. 8), *1265*] seldom, if ever, seen in other species [*860* (Ch. 8)]. Total estrogen excretion in patients with cervical carcinoma appears to be no different from the outputs of suitable control subjects (*1266*), but a relative excess of urinary estradiol and estrogen and deficiency of estriol has been claimed (*1267*). The eosinophile and karyo-pycnotic reactions in vaginal smears from women with cervical carcinoma were neither increased nor decreased, nor were they altered in women with uterine carcinoma (*1268*). In 19.6% of 459 pregnant women, Koga and Yamada (*1269*) observed abnormal cervical hyperplasia which disappeared in 85% in 6 to 24 weeks postpartum. In a study of cervical carcinoma patients and appropriate controls, Rotkin and King (*1270*) found no statistically significant correlations with several endocrine-related parameters such as age of menarche and menstrual disturbances, but claimed a higher frequency of abortions and "hormonal imbalance" in women with the disease. Estrogen therapy has proved ineffective in a small series with cervical carcinoma (*1271*); progesterone-induced improvements have been observed by Hertz *et al.* (*1272*) and their therapeutic significance denied (*1273*). A beneficial effect of Enovid has been seen (*1274*).

In a detailed study of cervical histology in 112 patients taking Enovid either cyclically or continuously. Hillemans *et al.* (*1275*) observed (a) partial regression of cells with anaplastic tendencies and (b) no progression of precancerous cells to genuine carcinoma, but no significant regression of such cells during the period of observation. Their conclusion is that the cytological effects seen resemble somewhat those seen characteristically in pregnancy.

Three deductions may be made from the foregoing: (a) hormonal control of cervical premalignancy seems to be quite possible, but once malignancy is established influence by ovarian hormones may be transitory; (b) the role of the complex endogenous hormonal milieu clearly demands thorough elucidation; and (c) therapy by synthetic steroids is an unknown area.

Mammary Glands and Lactation

The mammary glands are a prime target tissue for ovarian hormones. Both the growth of the mammary glands and the secretion of milk are estrogen and progestin conditioned. Estrogen generally stimulates duct growth and progestin lobule-alveolar growth. Lactation may be either stimulated or inhibited by estrogen depending upon dose and species or by estrogen plus progestin. It is not our province to describe in detail these basic hormonal influences and their variations which have been ably reviewed by Folley and his colleagues (*1276, 1277*). Our concern is with effects on breasts of fertility-controlling agents.

Since these agents have been administered almost exclusively to sexually mature women their effects on the pubertal growth of the breasts are not adequately established. Changes in breast size have been observed by users of these agents, but the available data suggest no markedly stimulative or inhibitory action at the usually employed dosages of estrogen-progestin combinations. This is illustrated in Table 62 which summarizes the responses to ques-

TABLE 62
EFFECTS OF ESTROGEN-PROGESTIN MIXTURES ON BREAST SIZE

| Drug | Dose (mg) | No. of subjects | Mean ± SE % with | | |
			No change	Increase	Decrease
Enovid	10	73	70 ± 5.4[a]	21 ± 4.8[a]	9 ± 3.4[a]
Enovid	5	383	87 ± 1.7	6 ± 1.2	7 ± 1.3
Enovid	2.5	164	80 ± 3.1	10 ± 2.3	10 ± 2.3
Ovulen	1–2	45	89 ± 4.3	7 ± 3.8	2 ± 2.1
Enovid withdrawn		61	82 ± 5.0	10 ± 3.3	8 ± 3.5

[a] ± standard error.

tioning concerning changes in breast size in users of oral contraceptives. The majority of subjects obviously note no change in breast size and those alleging decrease are just about balanced by those alleging increase except for the highest Enovid dosage where a fair proportion report some breast size increase.

Breast discomfort has been noted by some of the users of various oral contraceptives. This is complained of chiefly during the first cycle of use (*1109*) and the frequency of such complaints declines markedly thereafter. In Table 63 we present data taken from Wiseman (*1237*) on first cycle complaints. From 10 to 27% of users offer such complaint with no clear difference between the various preparations; however, women in postpartum lactation do not note any discomfort. Andrews and Andrews (*1161*) report moderate to severe breast soreness in approximately 6% of 340 Ovulen (1–2

TABLE 63

Reports of Breast Cycle Discomfort in First Medication Cycle

Preparation	No. of women	% with breast discomfort in 1st cycle
Enovid, 2.5 mg	686	13
Ovulen, 1 mg	102	22
Ovulen, 2 mg	100	10
Volidan, 4 mg	49	27
Orthonovum, 5 mg	43	26
Lyndiol, 4 mg	25	12
Enovid, 5 mg	49[a]	0
Enovid, 2.5 mg	48[a]	0.5

[a] Postpartum.

mg) users and slight discomfort in 34%. Mears (*1109*) observes similar incidences in Volidan users. These symptoms are probably referable to the action of the estrogen component on the nipple since Ferin (*1278*) has observed that with lynestrenol alone there was, if anything, a decrease in breast tenderness, whereas with lynestrenol plus mestranol there was a transient breast soreness in 29% of his subjects.

A number of observers have administered estrogen-progestin combinations to lactating mothers beginning at intervals varying from 3 to several weeks postpartum. We have presented data (Table 64) indicating that lactation tends to be diminished in subjects using higher doses of Enovid. Ferin *et al.* (*1279*) observed no significant effect on milk quality or growth rates of babies of mothers taking ethylestrenol or 6α-methylethynylestrenol. An apparent stimulation of lactation by these agents (*1280*) was disproven

TABLE 64

EFFECTS OF ENOVID ON LACTATING WOMEN (HUMACAO)

Dosage (mg/day)	Number followed up	% Lactating		
		Less than previously	Same as previously	More than previously
20	22	77	18	5
10	37	38	57	5
5	84	45	45	10
2.5	34	15	70	15

by the use of placebo tablets which stimulated the maintenance of lactation as well as the steroids.

Several of the steroidal agents used for fertility control have been used in the treatment of inoperable metastatic breast cancer [858, 860 (Ch. 8)]. Among them the 19-norsteroids have led to objective remissions in about the same proportion of cases as other effective compounds. This is indicated in Table 65 (1281) which indicates the ineffectiveness of oral progesterone but significant activity of norethisterone, methylnortestosterone, and norethynodrel.

TABLE 65

THERAPEUTIC TRIALS WITH ORAL STEROIDS IN BREAST CANCER

Compound	No. patients	% with objective remissions
Androsterone	22	4
Androstane-3α,17β-diol diproprionate	23	4
Androstane-3β,17β-diol diacetate	21	14
4-Androstene-3β,17β-diol diacetate	23	22
17α-Methyl-19-nortestosterone	21	24
17α-Ethynyl-19-nortestosterone	22	23
Progesterone	26	0
9α-Bromo-11-oxyprogesterone	25	20
Norethynodrel	20	20
Estriol-16α-methyl-3-methyl ether	25	16
2-Methyl-dihydrosterosterone	98	28
17α-Methyl-dihydrotestosterone	21	0
2α-Methyl-dihydrotestololactone	21	5
Testololactone	21	0
Δ¹-Testololactone	21	24

A 30% remission rate has been reported for advanced breast cancer patients taking oral norethisterone acetate (*1282*). Most of the remissions obtained with the steroids listed in Table 65 are transitory and the basis for the results observed is obscure. In rats, Huggins *et al.* (*1283*) find that a balanced progesterone-estrogen regimen will inhibit the carcinogenic action upon the breast of dimethylbenzanthracene. With a similar regimen clinical improvement has been observed in women with metastatic disease who have relapsed following adrenalectomy [*861* (Ch. 8)]. In contrast, medroxyprogesterone given alone caused hypercalcemia in 4 of 17 women with osseous metastases, suggesting exacerbation of the disease (*1284*).

The general concept that certain tumors of the breast are estrogen-dependent and that this dependence may be offset by androgens or progestins acting as estrogen antagonists still requires adequate experimental verification in man. Wilson (*1285*) has presented data suggesting the prophylactic action against breast cancer of estrogen and progestin in women, but extensive and careful statistical study is required to verify this thesis. Evidence for alterations in estrogen, androgen, or progestin metabolism in breast cancer cases has been sought with negative results (*1286*) or some suggestion of abnormality (*1287*). Indirect data on increased mammary cancer risk in pregnancy and lactation (*1288*) and on menstrual status as a prognostic factor (*1289*) encourage the belief in endocrine involvement. Further, the use of a discriminant function based on steroid excretion rates appears to differentiate women with breast cancer from cancer-free women of comparable age and condition (*1290*). Another discriminant function based on urinary steroid output (*1291*) appears to prognosticate the expectation of successful outcomes to ablative therapy or mastectomy. Application of this function to cases treated with steroids would be of interest.

Pregnancy and Postpartum

The action of the synthetic gestagens or of estrogen-progestin combinations in human pregnancy and parturition has been explored to only a limited extent. Possible effects on the initiation of pregnancy, i.e., fertilization and cleavage have been deduced;

thus Zanartu (*1242*) has observed luteal phase changes in postcoital cervical mucus specimens during the earliest days of cyclic use of several oral contraceptives (Anovlar, Lutoral, Lyndiol, and Enovid), only a few motile sperm on days 10 to 12 of medication and a complete absence of sperm on specimens taken thereafter. In contrast, Jackson (*1292*) found motile sperm in a normally liquid cervical mucus from Enovid users, but immotile sperm in a scanty mucus from Orthonovum users. Interference with pregnancy at the cervix would thus appear to be a possibility with certain agents.

What happens to sperm in the uterus and Fallopian tubes is another matter. In patients receiving Enovid immediately after "ovulation time," Rock and Garcia (*1293*) found no alteration in the conception rate compared to that of untreated control subjects. In a less well-controlled series, Tyler and Olson (*1294*) found an increased conception rate in patients receiving progestins and progestin-estrogen combinations and attributed this to replacement therapy in "inadequate" luteal phase. From these findings one might deduce that there is little probability that ovum cleavage or implantation is inhibited. On the other hand, the possibility of salvage suggested by Tyler and Olson is debatable. Hertig *et al.* (*1295*) found that only 42% of presumably fertile human ova survive to the twelfth postovulatory day; Vollman (*1296*) found that in 66% of 118 abortions occurring in 230 conceptions of normal healthy women, ovum loss occurred before or just after implantation. If progestin deficiency were the underlying cause of this loss a very high salvage rate should have been observed; indeed, faulty ova rather than faulty hormone production would appear to be involved in this large loss of early ova. Furthermore, Hertig (*1297*) has pointed out that decidualization occurs in the human after implantation so that this particular effect of the oral contraceptives may be premature.

The inhibition of abortion in women by gestagens or progestin-estrogen combinations is similarly a controversial subject. So-called salvage rates in habitual or threatened abortion rates have been challenged as statistically erroneous. For example, Meyerhof *et al.* (*1298*) found that weekly injections of 17-hydroxyprogesterone caproate to 18 women who had previously had only 17 normal deliveries in 72 pregnancies led to full-term deliveries in 15. But Shearman and Garrett (*1299*), using the same compound in a double-blind study with 50 women having a previous history of two or more abortions, found a 20% abortion rate in both the placebo and true medication groups; yet their data on pregnanediol excretion indicated that abortion occurred in those women with low outputs that failed to rise, i.e., due to progesterone deficiency. Osmond-Clark and Murray (*1300*) suggest that among such habitual aborters successful pregnancy may be predicted where the vaginal smear is normal and indicative of a normal hormonal milieu. In women with abnormal smears, gestagen treatment led to a salvage rate 33% higher than in untreated cases, although the latter received bed rest and sedation. Some evidence in a controlled study has been presented (*1301*) that salvage by oral preparations is most obvious with administration in the latter half of pregnancy.

The use of synthetic progestins in pregnancy has been challenged because of their masculinizing effects on the female fetus (*1302–1304*). As many as 18% of female infants born to 385 women treated with norethindrone were found to be somewhat virilized (*1305*). In contrast, an average daily dose of 400 mg of medroxyprogesterone acetate was given to 210 pregnant women and in the 108 female fetuses born there was no sign masculinization (*1306*). Yet at high dose in rabbits and rats this has caused pronounced fetal virilization (see page 170, Chapter 8).

Although large doses of progestins administered late in pregnancy have been found to suppress uterine activity (*1307*), a double-blind study with medroxyprogesterone acetate (20 mg 4 times a day) indicated no significant effect on the duration of pregnancy, on the characteristics of labor, or on fetal conditions (*1308*). The administration of Enovid or Provera at less than one hour postpartum prevented breast engorgement, pain, and lactogenesis with no other effect on the normal sequelae to parturition (*1309*). Apparently the estrogenic component was the primary inhibitor of engorgement, but the combination was essential for lactation inhibition. Transmission of synthetic steroids through the milk is suggested by significant skeletal advancement seen in 5 of 6 infants whose mothers were taking Pranone or Norlutin (*1310*) and gynecomastia in a male infant breast-fed by a mother using Enovid for contraception (*1311*). On the other hand, no signs of hormonal effect were seen in a large number of infants being nursed by Enovid users in Puerto Rico [*1133* (Ch. 11)]. Considerable amounts of corticosteroid but not of ovarian hormones have been found in cow and human breast milk (*1312*). A depot progestin (Provera) has been used to suppress menstruation in sexually precocious girls but with no other estrogenic or androgenic effect (*1313*). The suggestion of these data is that there are varying thresholds of response in children or that there may be coincidental occurrences of endogenous variations.

Functions Associated with Other Endocrine Organs

The effects of ovarian hormones upon the functioning of other glands of internal secretion have been discussed in previous chapters. The human does not appear to be exempt from some of the interrelationships observed in experimental animals. The two glands most studied have been the thyroid and adrenal cortex. Both tend to exhibit significant variation in function during pregnancy and in certain types of sterility. These interrelationships have been reviewed by Young [*740* (Ch. 8)] and Zarrow [*81* (Ch. 2)]. In this section we shall examine briefly reported actions of fertility-controlling agents.

THE THYROID

We have noted an increase in protein-bound iodine (PBI) in the blood of users of Enovid [*1091* (Ch. 11)]; this is illustrated in Table 66 where it may be seen that the increase is not dose dependent.

TABLE 66
PROTEIN-BOUND IODINE (PBI) IN ENOVID USERS

Daily dose (mg)	No. of subjects	PBI μg% Mean $\pm$ SE
Premed.	13	4.9 ± 0.41
2.5	63	7.9 ± 0.24[a]
5.0	127	7.3 ± 0.16

[a] Underlined values significantly different from premedication values.

A similar lack of dose dependency has been reported (*1314*) in the PBI increase seen with four oral contraceptives (Enovid, Orthonovum, Provest, and Lutoral). This increase in PBI and concomitant decrease in red cell uptake of triiodothyronine has been attributed to the estrogen component by Hollander *et al.* (*1315*), since

TABLE 67
COMPARISON OF AVERAGE THYROID UPTAKE
BEFORE AND 3 MONTHS AFTER DRUG INTAKE

	Mean ± SE		
	5 mg Enovid	1 mg Ovulen	2 mg Ovulen
No. of subjects	37	18	21
Before drug	19.6 ± 1.06	21.1 ± 1.22	18.1 ± 0.85
After drug	17.9 ± 0.93	19.7 ± 0.85	15.0 ± 0.64

medroxyprogesterone acetate given without added estrogen had no such effect. The PBI increase is attributable to the accompanying increase in thyroxine-binding globulin (TBG) (*1314*) which is also seen in pregnancy (*1316*) and during estrogen administration (*1317, 1318*). Norethindrone appears to increase thyroxine-binding

TABLE 68
COMPARISON OF AVERAGE THYROID UPTAKE IN LONG-TERM USERS
AND CONTROL GROUPS

Group	Enovid, 5 mg 3 yr and longer	Enovid, 2.5 mg, 3 yr and longer	Vaginal contraceptive users
No. of subjects	50	56	52
Average uptake	19.97 ± 0.59[a]	20.88 ± 1.07	20.94 ± 0.81

[a] Mean ± standard error.

prealbumin (*1314*). The increase in TBG does not appear to be progressive and the return to premedication values is prompt on discontinuance of oral contraceptives [*1091* (Ch. 11), *1314*].

In subjects studied before and after 3 months of use of two oral contraceptives, the data presented in Table 67 were obtained. They indicate a tendency to reduced radioiodine uptake by the thyroid of users of 2 mg Ovulen, but not by users of Enovid or

1 mg Ovulen. A comparison between long-term users of Enovid and vaginal contraceptive users presented in Table 68 indicates no effect on thyroid uptake of radioiodine. Maneschi *et al.* (*1319*) have, however, observed decreased I^{131} uptakes in euthyroid women taking 17-acetoxyprogesterone, its 6α-methyl derivative, and especially in those taking the combination of each with estradiol. They observed also hypothyroid-like effects on the globular and salivary indices. It should be noted that doses used were many times those used in simple therapy or for ovulation inhibition.

THE ADRENAL CORTEX

Adrenocortical ovarian interrelationships are indicated by such phenomena as increased circulating corticosteroids during pregnancy, the adrenogenital syndrome, and other disturbances in fertility seen in various types of adrenal hyperplasia.

The protective action of estrogen against stressful conditions and therefore the longer average life of women (*1320*) has been attributed to stimulation of adrenocortical secretion. On a daily output basis, women excrete less corticosteroid than men, but on the basis of mg per kg per day women's output values are no different from those of men (*1321*). The "protective" action of estrogen has been attributed to its stimulatory action on the reticuloendothelial system (*1322*). This would scarcely account for the antiarthritic effect of pregnancy which has been ascribed to an elevated tissue concentration of both cortisol and cortisone (*1323*). The reported remission of arthritis in women taking high doses (up to 30 mg per day) of Enovid (*1324*) has not been confirmed in a long-term study although a 50% reduction in the therapeutic dose of corticosteroid was observed (*1325, 1326*). A stimulation of endogenous corticosteroid secretion offers an obvious explanation of these observations. A clear stimulation of adrenocortical steroid excretion has been observed in men taking 100 or 200 mg per day of clomiphene (*1327*). The diminished carbohydrate tolerance observed in certain subjects taking Enovid (*1328*) may be attributed to the heightening of the glycosuric effect of cortisol observed on estrogen administration (*1329*) and noted in a diabetic woman taking Anovlar (*1330*). The reduced ACTH reserve noted in some of the Enovid users with reduced glucose tolerance (*1328*) and in subjects taking ethynyl estradiol alone (*1329*) suggests a possible direct action on adrenocortical secretion. However, we have been unable to observe any increase in cortisol production rates in long-term Enovid users. This is demonstrated in Table 69 where the mean production rates (based on isotope dilutions)

TABLE 69

CORTISOL PRODUCTION RATES IN
LONG-TERM ENOVID USERS AND CONTROL SUBJECTS

Months of Enovid therapy	Cortisol (μg/hour)
Control	412
Control	536
Control	493
Control	731
	543 ± 135[a]
93	540
59	294
104	460
94	861
	538 ± 238[a]

[a] Mean ± standard deviation.

for four Enovid users are seen to be identical with those for four matched controls. A direct corticoid action of medroxyprogesterone acetate has been demonstrated in adrenalectomized and hypophysectomized subjects (*1331*).

What does happen in subjects taking estrogens or progestin-estrogen combinations is an increase in plasma cortisol due at least in part to increased binding of cortisol to transcortin (*1318, 1332, 1333*). This is illustrated in Table 70 which demonstrates (a) the effectiveness of Enovid, its contained estrogen as well as its gestational component, and (b) the ineffectiveness of oral progesterone. The oral gestagen 17α-ethyl-19-nortestosterone alone administered to men has a mild effect on cortisol binding (*1334*). Since the half life of transcortin in human subjects is approximately 5 days whether estrogen treated or not it would appear that estrogen stimulates increased synthesis of transcortin (*1335*). Nonetheless,

TABLE 70

PLASMA CORTISOL IN PREGNANCY AND IN NONPREGNANT WOMEN
TAKING ORAL ESTROGENS AND PROGESTINS

Group	No. of subjects	Endogenous cortisol (µg/ 100 ml plasma)	% of Tracer dose of 7-H³- cortisol bound
Control	8	13.7 ± 4.3[a]	78 ± 3.7
Pregnancy, 3rd trimester	3	40.0 ± 1.8	86 ± 2.5
Enovid, 10 mg/day	8	30.8 ± 8.4	91 ± 1.5
Ethynylestradiol-3-methyl ether, 0.1 mg/day	5	24.0 ± 3.7	85 ± 5.1
Ethynylestradiol-3-methyl ether, 0.3 mg/day	5	32.0 ± 4.7	89 ± 2.1
Progesterone, 300 mg/day	5	7.5 ± 4.2	75 ± 3.0
Norethynodrel, 10 mg/day	5	25.5 ± 6.1	88 ± 3.6

[a] Standard error.

————Significantly different from control group @ 2% level of confidence ($P = 0.02$).

════════Significantly different from control group @ 1% level of confidence ($P = 0.01$).

TABLE 71

PLASMA CONCENTRATIONS (PC) AND METABOLIC CLEARANCE RATES (MCR)
OF CORTISOL IN LONG-TERM ENOVID USERS AND IN CONTROL SUBJECTS

Months of Enovid therapy	PC (µg/liter)	MCR (liters/hour)
Control	122 ± 15.9	3.4
Control	74 ± 5.7	7.2
Control	75 ± 12.5	6.6
Control	86 ± 5.9	8.5
Mean ± SD	89 ± 39	6.4 ± 2.2
93	280 ± 22.1	1.9
59	151 ± 17.5	2.0
104	154 ± 17.1	3.0
94	294 ± 18.9	2.9
Mean ± SD	220 ± 78	2.5 ± 0.6

TABLE 72

Urinary Steroid Excretion and Response to ACTH (80 U Intramuscularly) over 2 Consecutive Days in 4 Patients During Cyclic Enovid Treatment for 2 to 5 Years and in 4 Control Patients, Expressed as Mean Values ± S.E. in Milligrams per 24 Hours

	17-Hydroxycorticosteroids		17-Ketosteroids		Pregnanetriol		Pregnanediol	
	Enovid	Control	Enovid	Control	Enovid	Control	Enovid	Control
Prior to ACTH	[a]3.54 ±0.35	7.08 ±0.48	[a]4.90 ±0.71	7.21 ±1.16	[a]0.64 ±0.07	1.74 ±0.25	[a]0.73 ±0.06	1.42 ±0.27
Day 1 ACTH	19.01 ±3.23	21.33 ±2.30	12.12 ±3.09	16.52 ±4.03	2.48 ±1.40	5.34 ±0.82	0.94 ±0.01	1.90 ±0.18
Day 2 ACTH	22.94 ±3.05	22.82 ±4.26	17.09 ±0.93	22.74 ±7.84	4.96 ±1.52	9.95 ±2.64	1.44 ±0.39	3.40 ±1.02

[a] Values obtained by 15 separate determinations; other values are all based on 4 determinations.

as Table 71 demonstrates, the increased plasma cortisol in long-term Enovid users is accompanied by a reduced metabolic clearance rate. This might account for the increase in free plasma cortisol observed in men taking ethynylestradiol (1336) and certainly is consonant with the decreased excretion of 17-hydroxycorticosteroids in Enovid users [926 (Ch. 9)].

It is quite clear that adrenal responsivity to exogenous ACTH is not diminished in Enovid users (1337). This is illustrated in the steroid excretion response to ACTH administration observed in Enovid users and control subjects (Table 72). The ACTH-induced levels of urinary corticosteroids and 17-ketosteroids are clearly identical in Enovid users and control subjects. Urinary pregnanetriol and pregnanediol outputs tend to be less after ACTH administration to Enovid users, but there is considerable overlapping in individual values and the contribution from ovarian precursors cannot be assessed.

That adrenal malfunction may affect ovulation is suggested not only by the return to fertility of cortisone-treated women with adrenal virilism (1338) but by the ovulation induced by prednisone in less obvious cases of adrenal hyperplasia (1339). Here the inhibition of excessive ACTH secretion is the key to the restoration of a normal balance in pituitary tropic hormone secretion. The finding that small cortisone doses, presumably nonrepressive of ACTH, will produce ovulation in certain amenorrheic women (1340) suggests either a direct action on the ovaries or on hypersecretory adrenals.

Effects on Somatic Tissues and Functions

LIVER FUNCTION

Ever since the initiation of our large-scale studies with oral contraceptives, we have regularly undertaken liver function tests in our subjects [1090, 1091 (Ch. 11)]. In Table 73 are our data on the thymol turbidity test. Although the mean McLagen unit is significantly less in women taking various doses of Enovid and in those who have ceased taking medication (i.e., withdrawn), the percentage of abnormal values (outside the range 0.4 to 4.0 units) is highest in the premedication tests, almost as though the

TABLE 73

THYMOL TURBIDITY IN ENOVID USERS

Daily dose (mg)	No. of subjects	Mean ± SE	% Abnormal
Premedication	41	2.85 ± 0.25	9.8
2.5	154	1.46^a ± 0.10	0.6
5	373	1.67 ± 0.20	3.2
10	114	1.90 ± 0.26	2.6
Withdrawn	56	1.42 ± 0.13	0.0

^{a} Underlined values are significantly different from premedication values.

use of Enovid has tended to eliminate abnormal values. In Table 74, again in some instances we see significant mean difference between premedication values in the cephalin flocculation test and medication means. Here the percentage of abnormal values at 24 hours is about the same in treated and control groups.

In Table 75 are data on three other liver function tests taken before and after the use of Ovulen. Neither the transaminase nor the alkaline phosphatase values are significantly altered during medication, but the average sulfobromophthalein sodium (BSP) retention tends to be somewhat greater in the oral contraceptive users. In all forms of liver disease in man, hepatic BSP storage is reduced (*1341*). Increased relative hepatic storage of BSP has been observed in the last trimester of normal pregnancy (*1342*), after the administration of estrogens (*1343*), of various 17α-alkyl-19-

TABLE 74

CEPHALIN FLOCCULATION IN ENOVID USERS

Daily dose (mg)	No. of subjects	Mean ± SE		% Abnormal at 24 hr
		24 hr value	48 hr value	
Premedication	43	1.37 ± 0.24	1.64 ± 0.20	13.7
2.5	112	0.53^a ± 0.07	1.60 ± 0.08	4.8
5	293	1.15 ± 0.06	2.25 ± 0.08	15.7
10	146	0.70 ± 0.10	1.44 ± 0.13	11.6
Withdrawn	59	1.17 ± 0.15	2.07 ± 0.18	17.0

^{a} Underlined values are significantly different from premedication values.

norsteroids (*1344, 1345*), or of other anabolic steroids (*1346*). This effect on BSP metabolism appears to involve the excretory activity of the hepatic cell. In pregnancy and during the administration of the steroids the abnormal BSP retention is transitory and disappears with parturition or after cessation of drug administration. This reversible effect on BSP metabolism is not associated with abnormalities in conventional liver function test. However, in postmenopausal women taking Anovlar, Lyndiol or mestranol in rather high dose, BSP retention was associated with other signs of hepatotoxicity (*1347, 1348*), and a report of jaundice in three oral contraceptive users has also been made (*1349*). Swaab (*1350*) has

TABLE 75

LIVER FUNCTION TESTS IN OVULEN USERS

	No.	Premedication	No.	During medication
BSP retention (mg % at 45 min)	44	3.1 ± 0.40^a	32	4.9 ± 0.56^a
Transaminase (TransAc units)	46	12.3 ± 0.62	63	14.6 ± 0.98
Alkaline phosphatase (KBR units)	45	3.3 ± 0.10	62	3.7 ± 0.20

^a Mean ± standard error.

found normal blood bilirubin and SGOT transaminase in 500 Enovid (5 mg) users compared with nonusers. In some older women he has noted some irregularities. No laboratory or clinical evidence of hepatic dysfunction has been found in users of Lyndiol (*1351, 1352*) and in long-term users of several other 19-norsteroids no evidence of significant liver pathology has been found (*1353*). In a review of the effect of ovulation-inhibiting contraceptives on liver function, Arias (*1354*) states: "In summary, although ovulation-inhibiting oral contraceptives appear to affect hepatic cell excretory function, this effect is probably of little clinical significance. The available data suggest . . . oral contraceptives probably should not be given to patients with hereditary or acquired defects in hepatic excretory function." Haller (*1355*) concurs in the latter recommendation. Gellman (*1356*) finds no toxicity in 96 cases of accidental Enovid overdosage, including several instances where hepatotoxicity should have been evident if present.

Weight Gain and Aspects of Organic Metabolism

Weight gain has been reported occurring in users of oral contraceptives [cf. *1107, 1132* (Ch. 11)]. This is illustrated in Table 76 taken from Rice-Wray (*1357*). A significant percentage of patients taking Orthonovum (10 mg), Anovlar, and Lyndiol exhibited weight gain. A much lower proportion gained weight at the lower Orthonovum doses and no significant gain or loss is seen in Enovid and Lutoral users. Wiseman (*1237*) reports gains of 3 pounds or more in 34% of Enovid (2.5 mg) users, but 28% had

TABLE 76
WEIGHT CHANGE WITH ORAL PROGESTINS

Medication	No. of subjects	Percent		
		Gain	Loss	No change
Orthonovum, 10 mg	378	51.6	11.4	37.0
Orthonovum, 5 mg[a]				
Orthonovum, 2 mg	268	17.9	4.9	77.2
Noralestrine, 2 mg				
Enovid, 5 mg	201	4.5	12.5	83.5
Lutoral, 2 mg	303	13.5	12.6	74.9
Anovlar, 4 mg	504	30.5	16.3	53.2
Lyndiol, 5 mg	470	24.0	13.9	62.1

[a] This group began treatment with a 5 mg dose; the entire group was changed to a 2 mg dose.

losses of 3 pounds or more. Weight gains have been observed in diabetic postmenopausal women (*1358*) taking Enovid, but this may be associated with appetite changes or decreased sugar tolerance rather than with a protein anabolic effect as possible with the weakly androgenic gestagens, i.e., norethindrone, its acetate, and lynestrenol. A consistent association of high dosages of norethindrone with weight gain in an 8-month administration regime has been shown by Liggins (*1359*) even with added estrogen, whereas similar doses of 6-dehydro-6α-methyl-16-methylene-17-acetoxyprogesterone led to slight weight loss. Norethindrone acetate was similarly weight enhancing (cf. *1360*). As we have pointed out elsewhere, a probably important element in weight gain in oral contraceptive users is the loss of anxiety about accidental pregnancy with consequent appetite improvement. Furthermore, Mears, [1107 (Ch. 11)] has presented data on six oral contraceptives indicating that the percentage of patients showing weight gains of 3 pounds or over is maximal in the first 6 months to one year of use and thereafter declines.

There are relatively few studies of the action of fertility-controlling agents upon fat and carbohydrate metabolism. We have already mentioned the observation that the reduction in glucose tolerance seen in pregnancy is also observed in some women taking progestin-estrogen combinations. The explanation of this phenomenon is obscure. Since it occurs in a limited proportion of subjects, it may involve an "uncovering" of persons with a genetic tendency to reduced glucose tolerance or diabetes. As previously suggested, there may be involved an increased adrenocortical secretion through an estrogen-stimulated ACTH increase. Alternatively, estrogen may stimulate increased synthesis of an insulin-binding plasma protein.

The involvement of gonad hormones in fat metabolism has been the subject of study especially in view of the obesity of castrates of both sexes and obvious changes in depot fat in puberty and pregnancy. Some evidence has been presented that the loss of the anti-insulogenic action of gonad steroids may be responsible for the obesity of castrates (1361). In a review of lipid metabolism during pregnancy Scandrett (1362) points out that although estrogen administered to men reduces hypercholesteremia to normal levels pregnancy is characterized by an increase in serum lipids and in the β/α lipoprotein ratio. Since progesterone administration does not affect blood lipids (1363), the role of the ovarian hormones in fat metabolism in pregnancy is obscure. The therapeutic effect of certain estrogens in myocardial infarct patients [cf. 914, 915 (Ch. 9), 1364] has been attributed to their action in lowering blood cholesterol and β-lipoproteins.

Report has been made of a similar effect of Enovid administered at high dose to women with or without uteri (1365, 1366). In our premenopausal subjects we have observed no significant change in either blood cholesterol or β-lipoprotein levels following Enovid use at usual doses or the use of vaginal contraceptives (Table 77).

TABLE 77

BLOOD LIPID LEVELS (MG%) BEFORE AND AFTER USE OF ENOVID FOR
APPROXIMATELY ONE YEAR

| | Group | No. of cases | Levels[a] (Mean ± SE) | |
			Before	After
Cholesterol	Control	25	205.88 ± 7.971	194.12 ± 7.231
	Enovid	41	209.39 ± 5.288	200.07 ± 6.689
β-Lipoproteins	Control	25	2.64 ± 0.0868	2.37 ± 0.144
	Enovid	41	2.62 ± 0.0895	2.20 ± 0.415

[a] No significant differences were observed ($P > 0.05$).

This progestin-estrogen combination therefore does not in this respect imitate lipid effects seen in pregnancy.

Hematology

Some of the changes occurring in the blood and hematopoietic system during pregnancy have been attributed to the action of the increased circulating ovarian hormones (*81*). Thus the well-known anemia of the third trimester of pregnancy may be estrogen conditioned. It is characterized by a blood volume increase which has been induced in nonpregnant women by estrogen administration (*1367*); as a result the hematocrit falls, as do the erythrocyte and hemoglobin concentrations. Progesterone in experimental animals elicits an increase in total blood cell volume [*825* (Ch. 8), *1368*] so that it may balance the effect of estrogen. In Table 78 are presented data obtained before, during, and after oral contraceptive use in our subjects in Puerto Rico. Generally, these data confirm the expectation of the effect of a potent progestin tending to outbalance any putative estrogen action. Thus there is a rise in the hematocrit values of users and a tendency for an increase in the white cell count. Hemoglobin values show a significant drop at the highest Enovid dose and a significant rise in Ovulen (2 mg) users; the former may reflect the somewhat higher estrogen content or activity of 10 mg Enovid, the latter the potent gestagenic component of Ovulen. Enovid has been reported to suppress in normal women the usual midcycle fall in eosinophiles and leucocytes and the accompanying rise in blood platelet levels (*1369*), but otherwise no significant variation occurred in eosinophile or platelet counts and no thrombocytosis was observed.

During human pregnancy there is a progressive decrease in the total protein and albumin concentration in the blood and an increase in the globulins (1370). Certain 17-methylated androgens

TABLE 78

HEMATOLOGICAL DETERMINATIONS IN USERS OF ENOVID AND OVULEN

Daily dose (mg)	No.	Hematocrit (%)	No.	Hemoglobin (gm %)	No.	WBC/ml
Premedication	161	34.7 ± 0.34[a]	361	11.1 ± 0.08[a]	336	7,400 ± 105[a]
Enovid, 2.5	78	37.3 ± 0.44[b]	249	11.1 ± 0.06	303	8,230 ± 130
Enovid, 5	56	36.6 ± 0.37	333	11.1 ± 0.06	368	8,680 ± 270
Enovid, 10	—	—	85	10.6 ± 0.18	29	9,330 ± 480
Withdrawn	—	—	110	11.8 ± 0.17	116	7,680 ± 280
Ovulen, 1	84	36.9 ± 0.34	—	—	67	8,450 ± 356
Ovulen, 2	73	37.6 ± 0.45	26	11.8 ± 0.23	78	8,460 ± 270

[a] Mean ± standard error.
[b] Underlined values differ significantly from premedication values.

act to reduce blood albumin concentration and increase α-2 and β-globulin (1371, 1372). Enovid administration has led to a 21% depression in blood albumin concentration (1373), which is approximately the degree of depression seen in early pregnancy [81 (Ch. 2)].

The reported occurrence of thromboembolism in some users of oral progestin-estrogen combinations (cf. 1374) has led to some fairly intensive studies of coagulation factors in blood. The basic facts are as follows: (a) there is, on the average, a reduction in clotting time but no significant change in bleeding time in users—this is illustrated in Table 79, (b) there is an alteration in the concentration of certain clotting factors, but not of others—this is illustrated in Table 80 which demonstrates in Enovid users significant reduction over values for control subjects in mean prothrombin time (factor II), some increase in factor VII complex but not in specific measure of factor VII, an increase in fibrinogen (factor I) concentration along with an increase in fibrinolytic activity and no significant change in factors V (proaccelerin), VIII (antihemophilic), or factor X (thromboplastin-generating). Egeberg and Owren (*1375*) have found in Enovid users a shortening of cephalin time, some increase in factor VIII, and a slight increase in proconvertin activity. Turksoy *et al.* (*1376*) and Phillips *et al.* (*1377*) have found that estrogen, norethynodrel, and norethindrone will cause increases in blood fibrinogen, fibrinolysin, and antifibrinolysin. Sobrero *et al.* (*1378*) studying Orthonovum users could find no significant alteration in blood fibrinogen, in Lee-White clotting time, in partial thromboplastin time, in serum plasmin activity, or plasmin inhibitor activity. Pilgeram *et al.* (*1379, 1380*) in contrast find that Enovid users have increased profibrinolysin (plasminogen) and also an increase in plasma antithrombin. Brak-

TABLE 79

BLEEDING AND CLOTTING TIMES IN ENOVID USERS (CAPILLARY METHOD)

Years of use	No.	Bleeding time (sec)	No.	Clotting time (sec)
Controls	38	111 ± 8[a]	42	295 ± 9[a]
0–2	127	103 ± 4	127	246 ± 7[b]
2–4	102	116 ± 4	107	255 ± 8
4–6	17	148 ± 14	17	271 ± 12
Withdrawn	11	101 ± 18	11	276 ± 28

[a] Mean ± standard error.
[b] Underlined values differ significantly from control's.

man and Astrup (*1381*) reported in Enovid users no change in plasminogen or increase in fibrinolytic activity of isoelectrically precipitated euglobulins, but no development of inhibition of urokinase-induced fibrinolysin. Since this inhibition is seen in pregnancy they conclude that a faithful pseudopregnancy is not induced by Enovid. Since in pregnancy factors I, II, VII, IX, and X increase (*1382*) it is clear that pregnancy is varied from in users of certain estrogens, synthetic progestins, and progestin-estrogen combinations. Indeed, certain natural estrogens administered intravenously have no effect on clotting mechanisms except for a slight increase in factor V (*1383*), other estrogens may cause an increase in anticoagulant plasma mucopolysaccharides (*1384*), and estriol as a

TABLE 80
Enovid and Clotting Factors

Group	12 Controls Mean ± SE	5 Withdrawn Mean ± SE	P	8 Short-term[a] Mean ± SE	P	20 Long-term[b] Mean ± SE	P
Prothrombin, sec (II)	25.7 ± 0.58	26.0 ± 1.32	>0.9	24.0 ± 0.57	<0.05	23.8 ± 0.30	<0.01
VII Complex, sec	30.3 ± 0.64	29.4 ± 0.97	>0.4	28.2 ± 1.15	>0.1	25.2 ± 0.76	<0.01
Factor X, sec	30.8 ± 0.79	31.5 ± 0.80	>0.5	32.4 ± 1.18	<0.3	30.3 ± 0.61	>0.6
Factor V, sec	29.4 ± 0.79	30.9 ± 1.29	<0.6	28.4 ± 0.71	>0.3	30.3 ± 0.82	<0.5
Factor VIII, sec	82.5 ± 2.32	78.1 ± 5.40	<0.5	83.5 ± 1.91	>0.7	81.6 ± 1.69	<0.8
VII Specific, %	—	141.1 ± 28.78	—	122.4 ± 6.91	—	141 ± 8.80	—
Euglobulin lysis time, min	220.5 ± 10.15	160.4 ± 37.01	>0.1	87.8 ± 13.44	<0.01	146.3 ± 10.98	<0.01
Fibrinogen (I), mg%	357.2 ± 14.19	483.1 ± 42.07	>0.01	480.0 ± 28.57	<0.01	468.0 ± 14.10	<0.01

[a] Less than one year of use.
[b] More than one year of use.

succinate has a hemostatic effect in idiopathic thrombocytopenia (*1385*).

The suggestion of a possible hypercoagulability of blood in oral contraceptive users has been claimed as the basis for thromboembolic phenomena (*1375*), but Quick (*1386, 1387*) has questioned this on the basis of the variabilities in nonusers and the questionable role of coagulation factors in thrombophlebitis. Owren (*1388*) agrees that there is no proof of any causal relationship between

TABLE 81

DATA ON VARICOSITIES—ENOVID USERS AND CONTROLS EXAMINED IN PUERTO RICO AND HAITI

Daily dose (mg)	No. of patients	% with varices mean ± SE
Controls	63	49.2 ± 6.3
2.5	58	29.5 ± 6.0[a]
5	106	28.3 ± 4.5

Years of use	No. of patients	% with varices mean ± SE
0–2	63	49.2 ± 6.2
2–4	23	26.1 ± 9.2[b]
4–6	62	25.8 ± 5.5

[a] $P < 0.01$.
[b] $P < 0.05$.

thrombotic disease and the use of oral contraceptives; Swyer (*1389*) finds no evidence for a role of either estrogen or progestin in thromboembolism in women. These conclusions have been affirmed by the review by an expert committee of thromboembolic conditions in Enovid users and in nonpregnant women generally—no statistically significant difference in deaths from such conditions could be found and no meaningful correlates to the etiology of the disease (*1390*).

The increase in phlebitis in varicosities in pregnancy have also been attributed to hormonal action (*1391*) and found to have no hormonal basis (1392). Carey (1393) without offering any evidence states: "Oral contraceptives may occasionally stimulate the effect of pregnancy in aggravating varicose veins." In our examinations of Enovid users we found a lower incidence of varicosities than in nonusers. This is shown in Table 81, the data of which indicate that the longer term users have the lowest frequency of varicosities, perhaps a reflection of the long absence of pregnancy [1146 (Ch. 11)]. The hemostatic effect of 19-norsteroids in metrorrhagias (1394), menorrhagias, and other hypermenorrheic states (1395) may be marked by increased uterine vascularity and increased pelvic venous congestion (1396), but superficial veins do not seem to be target organs for these compounds.

Skin and Related Tissues

The effects of gonad hormones on skin pigmentation, spider telangiectases, hair growth, and acne vulgaris have been reviewed by Patterson (1397) and Kupperman [1069 (Ch. 10)]. The tendency to darker pigmentation in males is attributed to the action of androgen. It is interesting to note, however, that chloasma in women occurs during pregnancy and in certain darker skinned women taking oral contraceptives (1398). About 8% of 350 Enovid users in Puerto Rico have developed this condition (1398), and so did a higher proportion of Orthonovum users [1128 (Ch. 11)] perhaps because the Orthonovum contains a mildly androgenic 19-norsteroid. Androgen is presumably responsible also for certain types of hair loss (e.g., baldness in genetically conditioned men or women). We have questioned subjects using Enovid on hair loss with the results shown in Table 82. It would appear that there are less women complaining of hair loss and more alleging an arrest of hair loss among Enovid users than among control subjects.

Sebaceous gland development and sebum production as affected by gonad hormones has been reviewed by Strauss et al. (1399). Hamilton (1400) was among the first to indicate the direct acneogenic action of androgen in human subjects, the absence of acne in eunuchs, and its reappearance on androgen administration. On the basis of measurement of sebum production, Strauss and Pochi (1401) have found norethindrone and methandrostenolone to be androgenic whereas norethynodrel and 17-hydroxyprogesterone-17-caproate are not. Indeed they have found that Enovid causes a decrease in sebum production in women (*1402*), and is more effective than Ovulen or Norinyl (*1403*). The finding in a placebo-controlled experiment that prednisolone administered for 60 to 90 days caused the disappearance of acne in 50% of a group of mildly virilized women (*1404*) suggests a possible role of adrenal androgen, the production of which is suppressed by the corticosteroid. An occasional case of eczema seen in users of an oral contraceptive (*1405*)

TABLE 82
DATA ON HAIR LOSS—ENOVID USERS AND CONTROLS EXAMINED IN PUERTO RICO AND HAITI

Daily dose (mg)	No. of patients	% Alleging		
		A loss	Arrest of loss	No change
Controls	71	8.5	0.0	91.5
2.5	56	3.6	1.8	94.6
5	104	4.8	5.8	89.4

may reflect an allergic reaction to the contained steroids; estrogens on intradermal test in some women have given some evidence of such reaction (*1406*) as have other steroids [cf. Kupperman (*1069* in Ch. 10), p. 376 et seq]. Improvement in conditions with an allergic basis (e.g., asthma, eczema, vasomotor rhinitis) has also been noted (*1407*). A possible basis for certain reactions may be the role of estrogens in maintaining capillary strength in the skin (*1408*). Steroid hormones may be excreted through the skin (*1409*), and some of their metabolites may be odorful. Studies of these activities should be forwarded.

Psychological Effects

Effects of fertility-controlling agents upon emotional and behavioral phenomena are difficult to measure objectively. Thus the relief of migraine seen in users of certain 19-norsteroids (*1407, 1410*) may relate to loss of anxiety concerning pregnancy and not to an anti-allergic action. Psychiatric evaluations of 250 women

TABLE 83

THERAPEUTIC EFFECT OF ORAL CONTRACEPTION ON PREMENSTRUAL SYMPTOMS
(ETHYNODIOL DIACETATE, 0.5 MG WITH MESTRANOL, 0.1 MG)

Symptoms	Irritability				Depression			
	Before medication		After 3 med. cycles		Before medication		After 3 med. cycles	
	Patient numbers	Incidence (%)	Patient numbers	Incidence (%)	Patient numbers	Incidence (%)	Patient numbers	Incidence (%)
Severe or moderate	10/49	20	1/46	2	6/49	12	2/46	4
Mild	16/49	32	0.46	0	8/49	16	2/46	4
	26/49	52	1/46	2	14/49	28	4/46	8

taking Enovid demonstrated a definite improvement in sexual adjustment in most of them and no increase in emotional conflict or behavioral problems (*1411*). Again the roles of anxiety relief and suggestibility were not measured and it is notable that in a double-blind study with prednisolone and a placebo in oligomenorrheic women an equal proportion (60%) exhibited improvement in both groups (*1412*). One therefore regards with caution the reports of relief of psychotic disease in users of Enovid, although the relief of premenstrual tension may be involved (*1413, 1414*). The prevention of postpartum psychotic episodes by gestagens may be a direct therapeutic action (*1415*).

There seems to be little doubt that progestin-estrogen combinations relieve a number of symptoms associated with premenstrual tension (*1236*). This is illustrated in Table 83 by the data of Wiseman (*1237*) which demonstrates a marked drop in premenstrual irritability and depression in Ovulen users. Again, caution should be used in interpreting such data in the absence of a placebo control. This applies to the therapeutic use of other steroids, e.g., methyltestosterone (*1416*).

Libido and copulatory behavior are affected by the ovarian hormones. Although in primates copulatory activity may be maintained for long periods of time following ovariectomy (*1417*), the intensity and frequency of mounting, grooming, and allied behavior is markedly affected by estrogen replacement therapy (*1418*). In normal cycles sexual aggression appears to vary cyclically with ovarian secretory activity (*1419*). In women androgens appear to be potent stimulators of libido (*1420, 1421*) and in some instances progesterone has decreased libido (*1422*). On the basis of regular questioning we found no significant change in libido in Enovid users (*1423*). Records of the mean frequency of sexual intercourse showed, however, a tendency for an increase [*1090* (Ch. 11)]. Among Ovulen users this increased frequency appears to occur to a significant extent in the older subjects under study in Puerto Rico and at the higher Ovulen dosage (Table 84). Since the estrogen content is identical in the two dosages there is the suggestion that the progestin is the prime stimulator of increased coital frequency. Many other factors, e.g., freedom from anxiety, may be involved. The dissociation of the contraceptive act from the

TABLE 84

COMPARISON OF FREQUENCY OF COITUS PER MONTH BY AGE OF SUBJECTS

Contraceptive	20–24 Years		25–29 Years		30–34 Years		35–39 Years	
	No. of cycles	Mean ± SE	No. of cycles	Mean ± SE	No. of cycles	Mean ± SE	No. of cycles	Mean ± SE
Vaginal	—	—	454	10.0 ± 0.20	317	9.5 ± 0.17	299	8.44 ± 0.26
Ovulen, 1 mg	1289	10.3 ± 0.23	284	10.2 ± 0.28	56	8.9 ± 0.48	15	12.8 ± 1.10
Ovulen, 2 mg	1522	9.8 ± 0.11	706	10.3 ± 0.16	280	10.9 ± 0.22[a]	29	14.1 ± 0.55

[a] Underlined values differ significantly from vaginal contraceptive values.

sexual act has been considered an inducement to less restraint in coital enjoyment. In our opinion the possible psychological ramifications of fertility control have had most inadequate study. Some evidence that personality traits affect the way women use oral contraceptives has been presented (*1424*), but careful, adequately controlled objective studies of central nervous phenomena, aspects of behavior, and emotional reactivity are sadly lacking.

REFERENCES

1194. Layne, D. S., Meyer, C. J., Vaishwanar, P. S., and Pincus, G. 1962. *J. Clin. Endocrinol.* **22**, 107.
1195. Roland, M. 1958. *Ann. N. Y. Acad. Sci.* **71**, 638.
1196. Shearman, R. P. 1963. *Lancet* **I**, 197.
1197. Pincus, G. 1955. *In* "The Hormones" (G. Pincus and K. Thimann, eds.), Vol. III, p. 665. Academic Press, New York.
1198. Van Gansewinckel, A., and Ferin, J. 1958. *Bull. Soc. Belge Gynecol. Obstet.* **28**, 442.
1199. Lauweryns, J., and Ferin, J. 1964. *Intern. J. Fertility* **9**, 35.
1200. Schockaert, J. A., and Ferin, J. 1946. *Ann. Endocrinol.* **7**, 46.
1201. Laron, Z., Rumney, G., Rat, L., and Naji, N. 1963. *Acta Endocrinol.* **44**, 75.
1202. Taymor, M. L. 1964. *J. Clin. Endocrinol.* **24**, 803.
1203. Taymor, M. L., and Klibanoff, P. 1962. *Am. J. Obstet. Gynecol.* **84**, 1470.
1204. Schmidt-Elmendorff, H., Loraine, J. A., Bell, E. T., and Walley, J. K. 1962. *J. Endocrinol.* **25**, 107.
1205. Bell, E. T., Brown, J. B., Fotherby, K., and Loraine, J. A. 1962. *Lancet* **II**, 528.
1206. Rock, J., Garcia, C.-R., MacLeod, J., Pisani, B. J., and Southam, A. L. 1961. *Bull. N. Y. Acad. Med.* **37**, 689.
1207. Goldzieher, J. W., Rice-Wray, E., Schultz-Coutrerce, M., and Aranda-Rosell, A. 1962. *Am. J. Obstet. Gynecol.* **84**, 1474.
1208. Shearman, R. P. 1965. Symposium on Recent Advances in Ovarian and Synthetic Steroids. Sydney, Australia. (In press.)
1209. Peeters, F., Oeyen, R., and Van Roy, M. 1964. *Intern. J. Fertility* **9**, 111.
1210. Clyman, M. J. 1963. *Fertility Sterility* **14**, 352.
1211. Rice-Wray, E., Aranda-Rosell, A., Maqueo, M., and Goldzieher, J. W. 1963. *Am. J. Obstet. Gynecol.* **87**, 429.
1212. Pincus, G. 1959. *Studies Fertility* **10**, 3.
1213. Haman, J. O. 1942. *Am. J. Obstet. Gynecol.* **43**, 870.
1214. Greenblatt, R. B. 1959. *Clin. Obstet. Gynecol.* **2**, 232.
1215. Chalmers, J. A. 1959. *Proc. Roy. Soc. Med.* **52**, 516.
1216. Ferin, J. 1962. *Acta Endocrinol.* **39**, 46.
1217. Taymor, M. L., and Sturgis, S. H. 1961. *Obstet. Gynecol.* **17**, 751.

288   III. CLINICAL STUDIES

1218. Bernard, I. 1964. *Ann. Endocrinol.* **25,** 179.
1219. Klopper, A. 1962. *Proc. Roy. Soc. Med.* **55,** 865.
1220. Rice-Wray, E. 1964. *Proc. 7th Intern. Conf. Planned Parenthood, Singapore,* p. 358. Excerpta Medica, Amsterdam.
1221. Goldzieher, J. W., Henkin, A. E., and Hamblen, E. C. 1947. *Am. J. Obstet. Gynecol.* **44,** 668.
1222. Hisaw, F. L., Jr., and Hisaw, F. L. 1963. *Proc. Soc. Exptl. Biol. Med.* **114,** 486.
1223. Kistner, R. W. 1958. *Am. J. Obstet. Gynecol.* **75,** 264.
1224. Kistner, R. W. 1959. *Fertility Sterility* **10,** 539.
1225. Kistner, R. W. 1963. *Progr. Gynecol.* **4,** 319.
1226. Lebherz, T. B., and Fobes, C. D. 1961. *Am. J. Obstet. Gynecol.* **81,** 102.
1227. Riva, H. L., Kawasaki, D. M., and Messinger, A. J. 1962. *Obstet. Gynecol.* **19,** 111.
1228. Williams, B. F. P. 1962. *Am. J. Obstet. Gynecol.* **83,** 715.
1229. Mills, W. G. 1962. *J. Obstet. Gynecol.* **69,** 795.
1230. Palmer, R. 1964. *Intern. J. Fertility* **9,** 121.
1231. Williams, J. F., Williams, J. B., and Harper, J. 1962. *Am. J. Obstet. Gynecol.* **84,** 1512.
1232. Hvidt, V. 1962. *Danish Med. Bull.* **9,** 152.
1233. Wright, S. W. 1962. *J. Obstet. Gynecol.* **69,** 804.
1234. Linton-Snaith, R. 1962. *J. Obstet. Gynecol.* **69,** 799.
1235. Weinberg, C. H. 1957. *Proc. Symp. 19-Norprogestational Steroids,* p. 67. G. D. Searle & Co., Chicago, Illinois.
1236. Heller, C. G. 1957. *Proc. Symp. 19-Norprogestational Steroids,* p. 97. G. D. Searle & Co., Chicago, Illinois.
1237. Wiseman, A. 1965. Symposium on Recent Advances in Ovarian and Synthetic Steroids. Sydney, Australia. (In press.)
1238. Bishop, P. M. F., and Cabral de Almeida, J. C. 1960. *Brit. Med. J.* I, 1103.
1239. Bertrand, P., Dubreml-Fillman, Y., and Tonder, A. 1963. *Ann. Med. Nancy* **2,** 1011.
1240. Bishop, P. M. F. 1962. *Proc. Roy. Soc. Med.* **55,** 867.
1241. Borglin, N. E. 1964. *Intern. J. Fertility* **9,** 17.
1242. Zanartu, J. 1964. *Intern. J. Fertility* **9,** 225.
1243. Guard, H. R. 1960. *Fertility Sterility* **11,** 392.
1244. Frankel, P. A. 1961. *Intern. J. Fertility* **4,** 285.
1245. Beller, F. K., and Vogler, H. 1960. "Flow Properties Blood Biol. Systems," p. 248. Oxford, London and New York.
1246. Lee, L. E., Jr., Melnick, P. J., and Walsh, A. M. 1956. *Surg. Gynecol. Obstet.* **102,** 677.
1247. Pincus, G., and Garcia, C.-R. 1964. 16th Symposium del Cancer del Utero. Revista del Instituto Nacional de Cancerologica, Mexico City.
1248. Gore, H., and Hertig, A. T. 1962. *Clin. Obstet. Gynaecol.* **5,** 1148.
1249. Kaiser, R. 1959. *Arch. Gynäkol.* **193,** 195.

1250. Kelley, R. M., and Baker, W. H. 1960. *In* "Biological Activities of Steroids in Relation to Cancer" (G. Pincus, and E. P. Vollmer, eds.), p. 247. Academic Press, New York.
1251. Kelley, R. M., and Baker, W. H. 1963. *Progr. Gynecol.* **4,** 436.
1252. Kennedy, B. J. 1963. *J. Am. Med. Assoc.* **184,** 758.
1253. Bonini, L. D. 1962. *Ann. Obstet. Ginecol.* **84,** 420.
1254. Bonini, L. D. 1964. *Ann. Ostet. Ginecol.* **86,** 1.
1255. Toth, F. 1963. *Z. Geburtshilfe Gynaekol.* **161,** 94.
1256. Varga, A., and Henriksen, E. 1964. *Obstet. Gynecol.* **23,** 51.
1257. Mardones, E., Iglesias, R., and Lipschutz, A. 1954. *Proc. Soc. Exptl. Biol. Med.* **86,** 451.
1258. Griffiths, C. T., Tomic, M., Craig, J. M., and Kistner, R. W. 1963. *Surgical Forum* **14,** 399.
1259. DeWaard, F. 1964. *Nederl. Tijdschr. Geneesk.* **108,** 592.
1260. Rawson, R. W., and Rall, E. 1955. *Recent Progr. Hormone Res.* **11,** 257.
1261. Witherspoon, J. T. 1935. *Surg. Gynecol. Obstet.* **61,** 743.
1262. Hurxthal, A. L., and Smith, A. T. 1952. *New Engl. J. Med.* **247,** 339.
1263. Mixson, U. T., and Hammond, D. O. 1961. *Am. J. Obstet. Gynecol.* **82,** 754.
1264. Laffargue, P., Samso, A., Luscan, R., and Francois, H. 1963. *Ann. Anat. Pathol.* **8,** 85.
1265. Gardner, U. V. 1953. *Advan. Cancer Res.* **1,** 173.
1266. Murata, H. 1960. *Hirosaki Med. J.* **11,** 602.
1267. She, M. P., Lin, T. H., Chang, P. J., Cheng, F. L., Shen, C. Y., Lin, C. M., and Wa, A. J. 1963. *Chinese Med. J.* **82,** 475.
1268. Timonen, S. 1963. *Ann. Chir. Gynaecol. Fenniae* **52,** 143.
1269. Koga, K., and Yamada, M. 1960. *Kyushu J. Med. Sci.* **11,** 195.
1270. Rotkin, I. D., and King, R. W. 1962. *Am. J. Obstet. Gynecol.* **83,** 720.
1271. Nieburgs, H. E. 1953. *Obstet. Gynecol.* **2,** 213.
1272. Hertz, R., Cromer, J. K., Young, J. P., and Westfall, B. B. 1953. *J. Natl. Cancer Inst.* **11,** 867.
1273. Hertz, R., and Cromer, J. K. 1954. *J. Am. Med. Assoc.* **154,** 1114.
1274. Stoll, B. A. 1961. *Cancer Chemotherapy Repts.* **14,** 83.
1275. Hillemans, H. G., Ayre, J. E., and LeGuerrier, J. M. 1964. *Drug Res.* **14,** 784.
1276. Folley, S. J. 1960. *In* "Clinical Endocrinology" (E. B. Astwood, ed.), Vol. I, p. 518. Grune & Stratton, New York.
1277. Coure, A. T., and Folley, S. J. 1961. *In* "Sex and Internal Secretions" (W. C. Young, ed.), Vol. I, p. 590. Williams & Wilkins, Baltimore, Maryland.
1278. Ferin, J. 1964. *Intern. J. Fertility* **9,** 29.
1279. Ferin, J., Charles, J., Rommelart, G., and Beuselinck, A. 1964. *Intern. J. Fertility* **9,** 41.
1280. Ferin, J., VanCampenhout, J., and Charles, J. 1960. *Ann. Endocrinol.* **21,** 10.
1281. Segaloff, A. 1961. *Cancer Chemotherapy Repts.* **11,** 109.

1282. Curwen, S. 1964. *J. Endocrinol.* **28**, iii.

1283. Huggins, C., Moon, R. C., and Moril, S. 1962. *Proc. Natl. Acad. Sci. U. S.* **48**, 379.

1284. Kaufman, R. J., Rothschild, E. O., Escher, G. C., and Myers, W. P. L. 1964. *J. Clin. Endocrinol.* **24**, 1235.

1285. Wilson, R. A. 1962. *J. Am. Med. Assoc.* **182**, 327.

1286. Jull, J. W., Shucksmith, H. S., and Bouser, G. M. 1963. *J. Clin. Endocrinol.* **23**, 433.

1287. Gummel, H., Bacigalupo, G., and Schubert, K. 1960. *Chirurg* **31**, 491.

1288. Levin, M. L., Sheehe, P. R., Graham, S., and Glidewell, O. 1964. *Am. J. Public Health* **54**, 580.

1289. Kleinfeld, G., Haagesnsen, C. D., and Cooley, E. 1963. *Ann. Surg.* **157**, 600.

1290. Stern, E., Hopkins, C. E., Weiner, J. M., and Marmorston, J. 1964. *Science* **145**, 716.

1291. Bulbrook, R. D., Deshpande, N., Ellis, F. G., Hayward, J. L., Parker, J., Thomas, B. S., and Wang, D. Y. 1964. *Proc. Roy. Soc. Med.* **57**, 523.

1292. Jackson, M. H. 1961. *Proc. Roy. Soc. Med.* **54**, 984.

1293. Rock, J., and Garcia, C.-R. 1961. *Res. in the Service of Med.* **54**, 15.

1294. Tyler, E. T., and Olson, H. J. 1959. *J. Am. Med. Assoc.* **169**, 1843.

1295. Hertig, A. T., Rock, J., Adams, E. C., and Menkin, M. 1959. *Pediatrics* **28**, 202.

1296. Vollman, R. F. 1964. *Anat. Record* **148**, 347.

1297. Hertig, A. T. 1960. *In* "Les Fonctions de Nidation Uterine et Leurs Troubles," p. 169. Masson et Cie., Paris.

1298. Meyerhof, K. H., Brown, W. H., and Cioffi, L. A. 1962. *Current Therap. Res.* **4**, 499.

1299. Shearman, R. P., and Garrett, W. J. 1963. *Brit. Med. J.* I, 292.

1300. Osmond-Clark, F., and Murray, M. 1963. *Brit. Med. J.* I, 1172.

1301. Lee, K. 1962. *New Engl. Med. J.* **5**, 101.

1302. Wilkins, L. 1960. *J. Am. Med. Assoc.* **172**, 1028.

1303. Fine, E., Levin, H. M., and McConnell, E. L. 1963. *Obstet. Gynecol.* **22**, 210.

1304. Ishizuka, N. 1962. *Nippon Naibumpi Gakkai Zasshi* **38**, 443.

1305. Jacobson, B. D. 1962. *Am. J. Obstet. Gynecol.* **84**, 962.

1306. Goisis, M., and Cavalli, P. 1963. *Panmin. Med.* **5**, 107.

1307. Wood, C., Elstein, M., and Pinkerton, J. H. 1963. *J. Obstet. Gynaecol. Brit. Commonwealth* **70**, 839.

1308. Brenner, W. E., and Hendricks, C. H. 1962. *Am. J. Obstet. Gynecol.* **83**, 1094.

1309. Toaff, R., and Jewelewicz, R. 1963. *Lancet* **ii**, 322.

1310. Breibart, S., Bongiovanni, A. M., and Eberlein, W. R. 1963. *New Engl. J. Med.* **268**, 255.

1311. Curtis, E. M. 1964. *Obstet. Gynecol.* **23**, 295.

1312. Ratsimamanga, A., Mouton, M., and Bein, M. 1961. *Ann. Paediat.* **196**, 9.

1313. Kupperman, H. S., and Epstein, J. A. 1962. *J. Clin. Endocrinol.* **22**, 465.
1314. Florsheim, W. H., and Faircloth, M. A. 1964. *Proc. Soc. Exptl. Biol. Med.* **117**, 56.
1315. Hollander, C. S., Garcia, A. M., Sturgis, S. H., and Selenkow, H. A. 1963. *New Engl. J. Med.* **269**, 501.
1316. Peters, J. P., Man, E. B., and Heinemann, M. 1948. *In* "The Normal and Pathologic Physiology of Pregnancy." Williams & Wilkins, Baltimore, Maryland.
1317. Dowling, J. T., Freinkel, N., and Ingbar, S. H. 1956. *J. Clin. Endocrinol.* **16**, 1491.
1318. Carter, A. C., Feldman, E. B., and Wallace, E. Z. 1960. *In* "Biological Activities of Steroids in Relation to Cancer" (G. Pincus and E. P. Vollmer, eds.), p. 77. Academic Press, New York.
1319. Maneschi, M., Cittadini, E., and Quartararo, P. 1962. *Sicilia Sanit.* **4**, 135.
1320. Aschkenasy-Lelu, P. 1964. *Rev. Franc. Etud. Clin. Biol.* **9**, 109.
1321. Steeno, I., Menlepes, E., Hendrikx, A., Delaere, K., and Ostyn, M. 1963. *J. Clin. Endocrinol.* **23**, 677.
1322. Nicol, T., Bilbey, D. L. J., Charles, L. M., Cordingley, J. L., and Vernon-Roberts, B. 1964. *J. Endocrinol.* **30**, 277.
1323. Greaves, M. S., and West, H. F. 1963. *J. Endocrinol.* **26**, 189.
1324. Blois, J. A., and Demers, R. 1962. *Arthritis Rheumat.* **5**, 284.
1325. Rotstein, J., and Pincus, G. 1962. *Arthritis Rheumat.* **5**, 655.
1326. Gilbert, M., Rotstein, J., Cunningham, C., Estrin, I., Davidson, A., and Pincus, G. 1964. *J. Am. Med. Assoc.* **190**, 235.
1327. Morse, W. I., and Harkness, R. A. 1963. *J. Endocrinol.* **26**, xxviii.
1328. Waine, H., Frieden, E. H., Caplan, H. I., and Cole, T. 1963. *Arthritis Rheumat.* **6**, 796.
1329. Mestman, J. H., and Nelson, D. H. 1963. *J. Clin. Invest.* **42**, 1529.
1330. Paros, N. L. 1964. *Brit. Med. J.* **I**, 630.
1331. Cumanni, F., Massara, F., and Molinatti, G. M. 1963. *Acta Endocrinol.* **43**, 477.
1332. Laidlaw, J. O., Ruce, J. L., and Gornall, A. G. 1962. *J. Clin. Endocrinol. Metab.* **22**, 161.
1333. Metcalf, M. G., and Beaven, D. W. 1963. *Lancet* **i**, 1095.
1334. Apostolakis, M., and Tamm, J. 1962. *Klin. Wochschr.* **40**, 684.
1335. Sandberg, A., Woodruff, M., Rosenthal, H., Nienhouse, S., and Slaunwhite, W. R., Jr. 1964. *J. Clin. Invest.* **43**, 461.
1336. Marks, L. J., Friedman, G. R., and Duncan, F. J. 1961. *J. Lab. Clin. Med.* **57**, 47.
1337. Wallach, E. E., Garcia, C.-R., Kistner, R. W., and Pincus, G. 1963. *Am. J. Obstet. Gynecol.* **87**, 991.
1338. Wilkins, L., Crigler, J. F., Jr., Silverman, S. H., Gardner, L. I., and Migeon, C. J. 1952. *J. Clin. Endocrinol.* **12**, 277.
1339. Hochstaedt, B., and Langer, G. 1961. *Gynaecologia* **151**, 287.

1340. Jefferies, W. McK. 1962. *J. Clin. Endocrinol. Metab.* **22**, 255.

1341. Wheeler, H. O., Meltzer, J., and Bradley, S. 1960. *J. Clin. Invest.* **39**, 1131.

1342. Combes, B., Shibato, H., Adams, R., Mitchell, B., and Tramwell, V. 1963. *J. Clin. Invest.* **42**, 1431.

1343. Mueller, M. H., and Kappas, A. 1965. *Trans. Am. Assoc. Phys.* (In press.)

1344. Arias, I. M. 1962. In "Ciba Symposium on Protein Metabolism," p. 434. Springer, Berlin.

1345. Scherb, J., Kirschner, M., and Arias, I. M. 1963. *J. Clin. Invest.* **42**, 404.

1346. Marquardt, G. H., Fisher, C. I., Levy, P., and Dowben, R. M. 1961. *J. Am. Med. Assoc.* **175**, 851.

1347. Palva, I. P., and Mustala, O. O. 1964. *Brit. Med. J.* **2**, 688.

1348. Eisalo, A., Järvinen, P. A., and Lunkainen, T. 1964. *Brit. Med. J.* **II**, 426.

1349. Aldercreutz, H., and Ikonen, E. 1964. *Brit. Med. J.* **II**, 1133.

1350. Swaab, L. I. 1964. *Brit. Med. J.* **II**, 755.

1351. Linthorst, G. 1964. *Brit. Med. J.* **II**, 920.

1352. Rice-Wray, E. 1964. *Brit. Med. J.* **II**, 1094.

1353. Tyler, E. T. 1964. *Brit. Med. J.* **II**, 843.

1354. Arias, I. M. 1965. Communication to International Planned Parenthood Subcommittee on Oral Contraception.

1355. Haller, J. 1962. *Geburtsh. Frauenheilk.* **3**, 211.

1356. Gellman, V. 1964. *Manitoba Med. Rev.* **44**, 303.

1357. Rice-Wray, E. 1963. *17th Ann. Meeting Michigan Acad. Gen. Pract.*

1358. Cochran, J., Jr., and Pote, W. J., Jr. 1963. *Diabetes* **12**, 366.

1359. Liggins, G. C. 1965. Symposium on Recent Advances in Ovarian and Synthetic Steroids, Sydney. (In press.)

1360. MacDonald, R. R. 1964. *Practitioner* **192**, 834.

1361. Hausberger, F. X., and Hausberger, B. C. 1959. Abstract: The Endocrine Society.

1362. Scandrett, F. J. 1963. In "Human Reproductive Physiology" (H. M. Carey, ed.), Vol. I, p. 215. Butterworths, Washington, D. C.

1363. Oliver, M. F., and Boyd, G. S. 1956. *Circulation* **13**, 15.

1364. Stamler, J., Pick, R., Katz, L., Pick, A., Kaplan, B. M., Berkson, D. M., and Century, D. 1963. *J. Am. Med. Assoc.* **183**, 632.

1365. Cohen, W. D., Robinson, R. W., and Higano, N. 1961. *Circulation* **24**, 1087.

1366. Robinson, R. W., Cohen, W. D., and Higano, N. 1962. *Am. J. Med. Sci.* **244**, 736.

1367. Witten, C. L., and Bradbury, J. T. 1951. *Proc. Soc. Exptl. Biol. Med.* **78**, 262.

1368. Horger, L. M., and Zarrow, M. X. 1957. *Am. J. Physiol.* **189**, 407.

1369. Pepper, H., and Lindsay, S. 1963. *Am. J. Obstet. Gynecol.* **86**, 737.

1370. Mack, H. C. 1955. "The Plasma Proteins in Pregnancy." Charles C Thomas, Springfield, Illinois.

1371. Brennan, M. J., and Simpson, W. L. 1960. *In* "Biological Activities of Steroids in Relation to Cancer" (G. Pincus and E. P. Vollmer, eds.), p. 477. Academic Press, New York.
1372. McMath, M., Coon, W. W., and Block, G. E. 1961. *Cancer* 14, 1081.
1373. Pilgeram, L. O., and Pickart, L. R. 1963. *Proc. Soc. Exptl. Biol. Med.* 112, 758.
1374. Minogue, W. F., Halperin, I. C., Soler-Bechara, J., Varriale, P., and Flood, F. B. 1963. *New Engl. J. Med.* 268, 1037.
1375. Egeberg, D., and Owren, P. A. 1963. *Brit. Med. J.* I, 220.
1376. Turksoy, R. M., Phillips, L. L., and Southam, A. L. 1961. *Am. J. Obstet. Gynecol.* 82, 1211.
1377. Phillips, L. L., Turksoy, R. N., and Southam, A. L. 1961. *Am. J. Obstet. Gynecol.* 82, 1216.
1378. Sobrero, A. J., Fenichel, R. L., and Singher, H. O. 1963. *J. Am. Med. Assoc.* 185, 136.
1379. Pilgeram, L. O. 1964. *Brit. Med. J.* I, 883.
1380. Pilgeram, L. O., Amundson, B. A., and Lofgren, P. E. 1964. *Thromb. Diath. Haemorrhag.* 11, 94.
1381. Brakman, P., and Astrup, T. 1964. *Lancet* ii, 10.
1382. Phillips, L. L. 1963. *In* "Modern Trends in Human Reproductive Physiology" (H. M. Carey, ed.), Vol. I, p. 190. Butterworths, Washington, D. C.
1383. Wayne, L., Glueck, H. I., Brodine, C., and Coots, M. 1964. *Proc. Soc. Exptl. Biol. Med.* 116, 85.
1384. Roma, G. 1963. *Am. J. Obstet. Gynecol.* 87, 434.
1385. Polivoda, H., and Schmidt-Matthiesen, H. 1961. Proc. Congr. Soc. Haematol. 8th Art. 377.
1386. Quick, A. J. 1963. *Brit. Med. J.* I, 744.
1387. Quick, A. J. 1963. *Brit. Med. J.* II, 1604.
1388. Owren, P. A. 1963. *Brit. Med. J.* I, 1283.
1389. Swyer, G. I. M. 1963. *Brit. Med. J.* II, 808.
1390. The *Ad Hoc Committee* 1963. Final Report on Enovid for the Evaluation of a Possible Etiologic Relation with Thromboembolic Conditions. Food & Drug Administration, Washington, D. C. 1963.
1391. Goodrich, S. M., and Wood, J. E. 1964. *Am. J. Obstet. Gynecol.* 90, 740.
1392. Rivelin, S. 1962. *Brit. Med. J.* II, 547.
1393. Carey, H. M. 1963. *In* "Modern Trends in Human Reproductive Physiology" (H. M. Carey, ed.), p. 92. Butterworths, Philadelphia.
1394. Arrighi, L. A., Mendizabal, A. F., and Usubiaga, I. S. 1963. *Semana Med. (Buenos Aires)* 123, 1461.
1395. Rock, J., Garcia, C. R., and Pincus, G. 1960. *Am. J. Obstet. Gynecol.* 79, 758.
1396. Ryan, G. M., Jr., Craig, J., and Reid, D. 1964. *Am. J. Obstet. Gynecol.* 90, 915.
1397. Patterson, J. F. 1960. *In* "Clinical Endocrinology" (E. B. Astwood, ed.), Vol. I, p. 564. Grune & Stratton, New York.

1398. Esoda, E. C. J. 1963. *Arch. Dermatol.* **87,** 486.
1399. Strauss, J. S., Kligman, A. M., and Pochi, P. E. 1962. *J. Invest. Dermatol.* **39,** 139.
1400. Hamilton, J. B. 1941. *J. Clin. Endocrinol.* **1,** 570.
1401. Strauss, J. S., and Pochi, P. E. 1963. *Recent Progr. Hormone Res.* **19,** 385.
1402. Strauss, J. S., and Pochi, P. E. 1963. *Arch. Dermatol.* **87,** 366.
1403. Strauss, J. S., and Pochi, P. E. 1964. *J. Am. Med. Assoc.* **190,** 815.
1404. Goth, A., and Nenenfuhrer, L. 1964. *J. Clin. Endocrinol.* **24,** 1226.
1405. Carruthers, G. B. 1964. *Lancet* **i,** 981.
1406. Herschberg, A. D. 1960. *Rev. Ginecol. Obstet. (Rio de Janeiro)* **106,** 29.
1407. Mears, E. 1964. *Lancet* **i,** 981.
1408. Clemetson, C. A., Blair, L., and Brown, A. B. 1962. *Ann. N. Y. Acad. Sci.* **93,** 279.
1409. Klock, J. 1962. *Ned. Tijdschr. Geneesk.* **106,** 2204.
1410. Lundberg, P. O. 1962. *Acta Endocrinol.* **40,** Suppl. 687, p. 1.
1411. Zell, J. R., and Crisp, W. E. 1964. *Obstet. Gynecol.* **23,** 657.
1412. MacLeod, S. C., Morse, W. I., Hirsch, S., Tompkins, M. G., and Jacey, G. 1964. *Am. J. Obstet. Gynecol.* **89,** 642.
1413. Simpson, G. M., Radinger, N., Rochlin, D., and Kline, N. S. 1962. *Diseases Nervous System* **23,** 589.
1414. Swanson, D. M., Barron, A., Floren, A., and Smith, J. A. 1964. *Am. J. Psychiat.* **120,** 1101.
1415. Keeler, M., Kane, F., and Daly, R. 1964. *Am. J. Psychiat.* **120,** 1123.
1416. Kupperman, H. S., and Goodman, S. 1953. *Am. J. Obstet. Gynecol.* **65,** 141.
1417. Goy, R. W., and Eisele, S. G. 1964. *Anat. Record* **148,** 373.
1418. Michael, R. P., and Herbert, J. 1964. *J. Endocrinol.* **58,** vii.
1419. Rowell, T. E. 1963. *J. Reprod. Fertility* **6,** 193.
1420. Salmon, U. J. 1941. *J. Clin. Endocrinol.* **1,** 162.
1421. Greenblatt, R. B., Mortara, F., and Torpin, R. 1942. *Am. J. Obstet. Gynecol.* **44,** 658.
1422. Kupperman, H. S. 1961. *In* "The Encyclopedia of Sexual Behavior" (A. Ellis and A. Abarbabel, eds.), p. 494. Hawthorn Books, New York.
1423. Pincus, G. 1961. *Bull. Post Grad. Comm. Med. Univ. Sydney* **17,** 127.
1424. Bakker, C. B., and Dightman, C. R. 1964. *Fertility Sterility* **15,** 559.

CHAPTER 13

Some Consequences of the Application of Fertility Control

The Effectiveness of Contraception

The acceptability of methods of fertility control has been a widely discussed and rather controversial matter. It has involved primarily the acceptance of methods of contraception in various parts of the world or in various social and economic groups within a country or area. With advancing scientific knowledge, the traditional, folklore-based methods (*1425, 1426*) have given way to pragmatically proven methods of preventing fertility. It is not our province to review the history of the development of these methods and their socioeconomic interrelationships; such a historical review has been written by Himes and was recently revised (*1427*). Country-to-country variations in the use of various methods have been examined critically in a Symposium on Research in Family Planning (*1428*). As an illustration of some of the variabilities in the use of contraception we present Tables 85 and 86. The former shows the great variation from country to country in actual use of an effective contraceptive, while the latter illustrates the changes occurring in contraceptive practices within one country. The changes in practice are clear; the only method which has had a relatively unchanged proportion of users is the condom. With the advent of the oral contraceptives, a much greater change has probably occurred, but adequate statistics are thus far not available.

TABLE 85[a]

ANNUAL CONSUMPTION (DOMESTIC SALES) OF CONDOMS PER ADULT MALE
PER YEAR IN VARIOUS COUNTRIES

Country	Condoms per man per year
United States	11–13
Sweden	10
Japan	8
United Kingdom	5
West Germany	5
Hungary	3
France	1
India	0.06

[a] From Tietze (1429).

Acceptability of one method or another would seem therefore to vary with national culture patterns [e.g., the use of abortion (1431) in Japan] and perhaps to a lesser extent with the actual effectiveness of a method.

In this connection it is interesting to compare the data of Table 86 with those of Table 87, which present the pregnancy rates for

TABLE 86

THE FREQUENCY OF USE OF VARIOUS CONTRACEPTIVE METHODS
IN THE UNITED STATES

Method	% in 1936 (1427)	% in 1955 (1430)
Withdrawal	29	7
Douche	26	7
Condom	24	26
Diaphragms	3	24
Others	17	15
Rhythm		21

various contraceptive methods. They indicate some correlation between the most efficient methods and the proportion of users in 1955. In a comparative study of three barrier methods in low socioeconomic groups, Dingle and Tietze (1434) found pregnancy rates of 14.5 for the diaphragm, 24.0 for spermicidal jelly alone, and 22.5 for foam tablets. These data are not too different from those of Table 87. Frank (*1435*) reports a rate of 23.1 for a vaginal jelly used by clinic patients in Chicago. In Ceylon a rate of 20 was found among users of a foam tablet (*1436*). These very similar rates for users of a given method in various areas suggest a similarity of effectiveness which may not be related to carelessness in use which is the commonly held cause of undesired pregnancies.

When consideration is given to more modern methods of contraception two emerge as highly effective: oral contraception and the use of intrauterine devices (IUCD). The pregnancy rates in

TABLE 87

PREGNANCY RATES PER 100 YEARS OF EXPOSURE
FOR VARIOUS METHODS OF CONTRACEPTION

Method	Data for American families (*1432*)	Data by Venning from six sources (*1433*)
Condom	13.8	14
Diaphragm	14.4	12
Withdrawal	16.8	18
Rhythm	38.5	24
Douche	40.5	31
Jelly alone	—	20
All other[a]	30.3	—

[a] Including combined and alternate use.

users of IUCD vary from 0.9 per 100 woman years in users of stainless steel rings (*1437*) to 8.5 in users of silver rings (*1438*). The use of spiral plastic IUCD has been similarly effective with pregnancy rates of 5.1 (Margulies spiral), 4.5 for Lippes loop wearers in the United States (*1439*), and 7.5 for wearers in Humacao, Puerto Rico (*1440*). With increased use and experience, pregnancy rates in users of IUCD tend to be rather similar to those for users of various other devices (*1441*). A complicating factor is the expulsion, often unnoticed, of IUCD. Such expulsions may vary, depending on the device, from 0 to 20% in a year and continue to occur at a regular rate in many instances (*1441*). Reinsertions are accepted in a number of cases. Objects which cannot be expelled through the cervix and vagina may be extruded through the uterine wall into the abdominal cavity. In a review of studies with certain

IUCD (Margulies spirals and Lippes loops), Kirckhoff and Haller (*1442*) list 15 objections to their use, e.g., the occurrence of spotting, metrorrhagia, menorrhagia, various reproductive tract infections, danger of carcinoma. In contrast, advocates of their use find the only contraindications to be pregnancy, large fibromyomas, cervicitis (or other pre-existing infection), and adnexal disease (*1439*). Acceptance has been intensified in some areas, e.g., Taiwan (*1443*), by "action programs." Rejection rates are not accurately known, but Zipper *et al.* (*1444*) have reported discontinuance by 20% of users during a 15-month period of a flexible Nylon ring, and Tietze and Lewit (*1441*) report 11% of IUCD removed for medical and 2% for personal reasons in the first year of use.

IUCD are now on trial in a number of countries including Hong Kong, Taiwan, India, Korea, Chile, Jamaica, Fiji, Malaysia, Denmark, Japan, Southern Rhodesia, and the United States (*1445*). The mechanism of their action is not established—in rats they affect ovum transport, in rabbits implantation and postimplantation stages are affected, in cows ovum expulsion due to hyperestrinism occurs, and in monkeys tubal ova are lost (*1445*). A general explanation might be a reflex stimulation of processes leading to excess ovarian estrogen or increased sensitivity of the uterus to estrogen (*1446*). Since implantation and pregnancies have occurred in some women with IUCD *in situ*, the problem of mechanism in the human is difficult. Data on possible physiological effects of IUCD are lacking. There are no studies on possible hematological effects, liver function changes, ovarian responses, endocrine alterations, etc., etc. Inflammatory responses due to their insertion have occurred in the uteri in 36% of users in Hong Kong (*1447*), but no abnormal endometrial histology was seen in users in New York City (*1448*). It is therefore difficult to understand the undesirable complications listed by Saigal (*1449*). It is obvious that careful, objective, controlled studies of many physiological functions are needed.

The Acceptability of Contraception

Contraceptive effectiveness of oral progestin-estrogen combinations is clearly greater than that for any other method. In our early studies we found a pregnancy rate of 1.1 per 100 woman years (Table 40), which in allegedly faithful users fell to 0.2 (Table 41).

In a contraceptive clinic in Slough in England [*1237* (Ch. 12)], the rate in initial trials was 1.0 and in recent years the failure rate was 0.1%. The previous failure rate in women in this same clinic was 33% for users of diaphragms, 50% in cases where condoms were used, 74% in users of vaginal chemical contraceptives, and 100% in those practising coitus interruptus, with an overall failure rate of 40%. In this clinic the use of oral contraceptives was initiated in 1962 when 19% of patients requested them, in 1963 51% were using them and during the first half of 1964 this proportion rose to 75%, and this despite much publicity given to possible dangers in the

TABLE 88

COMPARATIVE STUDY

Contraceptive	No. at start	% Remaining after		
		1 Year	2 Years	2½ Years
Enovid, 2.5 mg	199	57.9	28.2	18.6
Orthonovum, 2 mg	194	65.1	31.8	18.0
Ovulen, 1 mg	164	61.0	19.3	8.3

use of this medication. With the increase in the recruitment rate, there has been a decrease in the drop-out rate. In a group of problem patients followed for 5 years in another clinic in England, the failure rate for women taking oral contraceptives was 7.3, whereas among these women the rates for condom use and diaphragm use were 27.7 and 40, respectively. In Madras 74% of patients entering a trial study with Enovid (2.5 mg) dropped out within the year [*1147* (Ch. 11)]. Elsewhere drop-out rates were much less, e.g., 6% in Holland [*1164* (Ch. 11)], 17% in Mexico [*1220* (Ch. 12)], 8 to 20% in London (*1450*), 28% in Singapore (*1450a*).

In Humacao, Puerto Rico, a comparative study of three oral preparations has been in progress for 3 years. Equal numbers of women were recruited at first for Enovid and Orthonovum trials, and a somewhat lower number for Ovulen trials which had begun a few months later. In Table 88 are listed the numbers involved and the rate of loss of users of these three drugs. In 2½ years 82 to 92% of those starting were no longer using the drugs. When the reasons for discontinuing are catalogued (Table 89), it may be seen that

TABLE 89

COMPARATIVE STUDY—REASONS FOR DISCONTINUING

Reasons	Enovid (142)[a]	Orthonovum (121)	Ovulen (107)
1. Contraception abandoned	14.8	11.6	15.0
2. Changed method	13.4	11.6	8.4
3. Reactions to drug	27.4	21.5	21.5
4. Moved away or not contacted	10.6	12.4	17.7
5. Husband opposed	2.1	3.3	1.9
6. Contraception not needed	16.9	24.0	21.5
7. Propaganda	6.3	2.5	3.6
8. Planning pregnancy	8.5	13.2	8.4
9. Miscellaneous	0.0	0.0	1.9

[a] Number questioned.

rejection of the drug (item 3) was involved in 21.5 to 27.4% of those leaving the study. Those returning to presumably normal chances of exposure to conception totaled 50.4 to 59.1% of those leaving (items 1, 3, 5, 7, and 8). In Table 90 are listed the reasons for discontinuance proferred by the users of Enovid and Ovulen. It

TABLE 90

COMPARISON OF REASONS FOR LEAVING GIVEN BY SUBJECTS
IN SAN JUAN, PUERTO RICO

Reasons	293 Enovid users (1957–1960) (%)	153 Ovulen users (1961–1964) (%)
Reactions	28	10
No interest	11	36
Moved	14	10
Sterilized (husband or wife)	12	3
Separated	9	6
Unrelated illness	5	4
Propaganda against	5	0
Pregnant during use	4	3
Wanting another child	3	4
Afraid	3	3
Husband opposed	3	1
Miscellaneous	2	4
Uncooperative	0	17

will be seen that objections to side effects of the drug (reactions) are much less in those leaving the Ovulen trials than in those that left the Enovid trial. "No interest" and "uncooperative" are the chief causes of abandonment, but these categories may indicate interreactions of the project supervisor with the volunteers. In brief, motivation for abandoning contraception may be quite varied and a function of the project site, management, and drug used.

If we examine in detail the reasons for abandoning oral contraception, we find that the one particularly associated with the estrogen-progestin medication is unpleasant side effects including

TABLE 91

COMPARATIVE STUDY OF TYPES OF COMPLAINT (%/CYCLE) IN ENOVID (EN), ORTHONOVUM (OR), AND OVULEN (OV) USERS

Complaints	Cycles 1–3			Cycles 12–14			Cycles 25–27		
	En	Or	Ov	En	Or	Ov	En	Or	Ov
Gastric symptoms	15	10	11	10	5.3	4.2	0.6	3.7	3.8
Headache and dizziness	13	11	9	10	14	12	5.0	3.2	8.9
Nervousness, weakness, and malaise	5.8	4.0	1.9	3.6	3.2	2.9	0.0	3.9	0.6
Total % of complaints	33.8	25.0	21.9	23.6	22.5	19.1	5.6	10.8	13.3

gastric symptoms such as nausea, gastralgia, or sometimes vomiting, headache, and dizziness and nervousness, weakness, or malaise. These "reactions" to the use of these drugs tend to be maximal in early cycles of use and to decline in frequency and severity thereafter. This has been reported in practically all investigations or oral contraceptives. It is illustrated in the data of Table 91 which gives the percent per cycle of these types of complaint in the first three, the 12th to 14th and the 25th to 27th cycles of use of three preparations administered in the comparative study mentioned above. There is a marked drop, particularly in the frequency of some gastric symptoms, in the users of each preparation. Headache and dizziness, which are rather common menstrual occurrences, declined less markedly in incidence, and the proportion with nervousness, etc., did not change significantly in Orthonovum users but did fall off in Enovid and Ovulen users.

Because of the greater frequency of the "reactions" in early cycles we suspected a psychogenic basis, i.e., a reflection of apprehension due to the use of a new and unfamiliar method of contraception, the fact that the nurse or social worker requested an accounting of all untoward events during the cycle, and so on. We therefore initiated in Puerto Rico an experiment in which to two groups of women using conventional contraceptives there were assigned on a random basis tablets A or B identical in size and

TABLE 92

EFFECTS OF NO ADMONITION AND PLACEBOS VERSUS TRUE MEDICATION
ON MENSTRUAL CYCLE PHENOMENA

Group	No. of subjects	No. of cycles	Mean length (days)	% with Reactions	Breakthru	Amenorrhea
No admonition	15	48	29.2	6.3 ± 3.5^a	2.1 ± 2.1^a	0.0^a
Placebo	15	41	31.6	17.1 ± 5.9	4.9 ± 3.2	9.8
True medication	13	30	25.5	23.3 ± 7.7	16.7 ± 6.8	3.3

$^a \pm$ standard error.

appearance. The A tablets contained the progestin-estrogen mixture (Enovid, 10 mg), while the B tablets contained lactose, but neither the social worker distributing them nor the physician-in-charge knew which was which. The volunteer subjects, of course, knew no difference, and were told not to abandon their usual contraceptives as they were being "tested" as possible beneficiaries of oral contraception and all symptoms were to be noted. Regular monthly visits and questioning concerning complaints were carried on as usual for a 3- to 4-month period. At the same time in a city 40 miles away from that in which the A and B tablet receivers lived we offered Enovid (10 mg) to a group of subjects with no admonition concerning possible "reactions." At the monthly visit, inquiry concerning complaints were also made. In Table 92 are the data on the three groups. The higher incidence (23.3%) of "reactions" in the users of the true medication is not significantly different from that observed in the placebo users (17.1%), but is significantly higher than the incidence in the no admonition subjects (6.3%). These data speak for themselves as a commentary on the eliciting of subjective data. They illustrate the need for carefully controlled observations stressed by Beecher (*1451*) for drug studies generally and by Puddy (*1452*) specifically for oral contraceptive studies.

The "reactions" are, of course, mostly real and not simulated. Furthermore, a small proportion of them may indeed involve the effects of a transition from a woman's characteristic ovarian hormone controlled cyclic events to those instituted by exogenous hormone control. Nonetheless, most of them are not reflective of physiological actions of the drugs. This is illustrated by two sets of data presented in Tables 93 and 94. The patients entering a study

TABLE 93
ONE-HUNDRED TWENTY-TWO PATIENTS TAKING OVULEN QUESTIONED
CONCERNING UNDESIRABLE MENSTRUAL SYMPTOMS ("REACTIONS")

"Reactions"	Number	%
None before or during medication	45	37
None before, but some during medication	29	24
Before and during medication	20	16
Before, but none during medication	28	23
Therefore, % "cured" of reactions: 58.4	$\left(\dfrac{28}{28+20}\right)$	
Therefore, % with induced reactions: 39.2	$\left(\dfrac{29}{29+45}\right)$	

with Ovulen were questioned as to the occurrence of gastric symptoms, headaches, dizziness, nervousness, etc., in their menstrual cycles. Every complaint of such symptoms during Ovulen use was recorded. The results presented in Table 93 indicate that 60% of the women reported no "reactions" during medication, whereas 40% did. The failure of "reactions" to appear in subjects previously having them might be considered a "cure" effected by the medication, i.e., in 58.4%, whereas the occurrence of such symptoms during medication in patients having none previous to drug use could be considered an "induction" of these symptoms by the drug i.e., 39.2%. Actually the before and after occurrences are probably random events not related to the medication.

In Table 94 we list the percentage of the patients using Enovid from 1957 to 1960 who withdrew from our studies because of "reactions"; a similar tabulation is made for Ovulen users leaving during 1961 to 1964. It is clear that Ovulen users presented this as a reason for leaving much less frequently than Enovid users. It should be noted, however, that the Enovid users were the pioneers in a novel method. In brief, factors unrelated to the physiology of oral contraception may figure importantly in the statistics of their use. These factors may involve propaganda, the culture patterns

TABLE 94

THE PERCENTAGE OF SUBJECTS ABANDONING ORAL CONTRACEPTION BECAUSE OF "REACTIONS"

Contraceptive	In 1st year	In 2nd year	In 3rd year
Enovid	13.8	4.3	3.2
Ovulen	5.1	2.9	1.9

of a particular group, public confidence or publicity "scares," interpersonal relations between project supervisors and volunteers, the degree of understanding of the biology of the method, and so on.

One factor in acceptability and use has been much discussed. This is the socioeconomic status of the women. The data of Rice-Wray (1453) presented in Table 95 are quite illuminating on this point. They demonstrate a minimum rate of dropping out in the poorest subjects and a maximal incidence in the well-to-do. The occurrence of "reactions" was similar in all the five groups of Table 95. Rice-Wray believes: "that an upper class woman is less willing to accept nausea or headache even for a cycle or two" whereas "poor women are so desperate at the thought of an unwanted pregnancy that they are willing to accept some discomfort in order to be safe." That this may not be a complete explanation is suggested by the data of Peberdy, cited by Mears [1107 (Ch. 11)], on problem women who had quite high pregnancy rates when allegedly using diaphragms (40 per 100 woman years) or condoms (28 per 100 woman years) but a much lower rate with oral con-

Onuma, H., 169(837), *181*(837)
Orias, O., 201(978), *213*(978)
Orsini, M. W., 114(527), 116(539), *145*(527, 539)
Ortavant, R., 191(932), *195*(932)
Osborn, F., 305(1458), *307*(1458)
Osenkoop, R. S., 15(59), *25*(59)
Osima, B., 81(339, 343), *86*(339, 343)
Oslapas, R., 74(293), *85*(293)
Oslund, R. M., 44, *49*
Osmond-Clark, F., 265(1300), *290* (1300)
O'Steen, W. K., 78(314), *85*(314)
Ostyn, M., 268(1321), *291*(1321)
Overbeek, G. A., 73(288), *164* (768), 85(288), *179*(768)
Owren, P. A., 279(1375), 281(1375, 1388), *293*(1375, 1388)
Ozawa, M., 211(1071), *216*(1071)

P

Pagani, C., 223(1120), *233*(1120)
Paget, G. E., 35(133), 232(133), *54*(133)
Palka, Y. S., 73(283), *84*(283)
Pallos, K. V., 29(106), *53*(106)
Palm, J., 98(442), *101*(442)
Palmer, R., 250(1230), *288*(1230)
Palva, I. P., 274(1347), *292*(1347)
Paniagua, M., 219(1088, 1089), *232* (1088, 1089)
Panse, T. B., 140(623), *148*(623)
Papanicolaou, G. N., 200(976), *213* (976)
Papatheodorou, B., 35(123), *54*(123)
Pappo, R., 166(784), *179*(784)
Papworth, R. A., 227(1136), *234* (1136)
Paredis, F., 96(430), *101*(430)
Parizek, J., 36(138), *54*(138)
Parke, J. A. C., 200(972), *212*(972)
Parker, J., 263(1291), *290*(1291)
Parkes, A. S., 18(72), 19(75), 93 (395), 105(468), 141(630, 632),

232(1193), 25(72, 75), *100*(395), *109*(468), *148*(630, 632), *235* (1193)
Parlow, A. F., 73(287), 205(1021), 229(1021), 85(287), *214*(1021)
Paros, N. L., 268(1330), *291*(1330)
Parsons, E. I., 42, 95(416), *49, 101* (416)
Partington, M., 104(463), *109*(463)
Pasteels, J. L., 57(210), *82*(210)
Patanelli, D. J., 29(111), 37(153, 155, 156), 53(111), 55(153, 155, 156)
Patterson, J. F., 282(1397), *293* (1397)
Patwardhan, V. V., 140(623), *148* (623)
Paul, H. E., 37(148), *55*(148)
Paul, M. F., 37(148), *55*(148)
Paulsen, C. A., 189(924, 928, 929), 192(941), 195(924, 928, 929), *196* (941)
Paulson, E., 143(650), 171(856), *148*(650), *181*(856)
Pean, V., 219(1089), *232*(1089)
Pearse, J. J., 81(342), *86*(342)
Pecile, A., 71(257), 73(281), 118 (552), 84(257, 281), *146*(552)
Peeters, F., 228(1151), 243(1209), 234(1151), *287*(1209)
Pendleton, A., 219(1089), *232*(1089)
Pennefeather, J. N., 143(652), *149* (652)
Pennell, R. B., 210(1063), *215* (1063)
Pepper, H., 277(1369), *292*(1369)
Perey, B., 12(39), *24*(39)
Perez-Vega, E., 223(1115), *243* (1115), *233*(1115)
Perlbachs, M., 82(361), *87*(361)
Pernot, E., 43, 45, *49*
Perrine, J. W., 68(249), *83*(249)
Persico, M., 168(819), *181*(819)
Pesch, L. A., 169(831), *181*(831)
Peters, J. P., 267(1316), *291*(1316)

Simpson, E. C., 166(793), *180*(793)
Simpson, G. M., 285(1413), *294*
(1413)
Simpson, M. E., 11(35), 18(70, 71),
80(337), *24*(35), *25*(70, 71), *86*
(337)
Simpson, W. L., 278(1371), *293*
(1371)
Singer, B., 169(823), *180*(823)
Singher, H. O., 279(1378), *293*
(1378)
Skrebnik, H. H., 144(659), *149*(659)
Slaunwhite, W. R., Jr., 269(1335),
291(1335)
Slechta, R. G., 6(24), 103(24), *9*
(24)
Sloan, S. H., 157(713), 159(731),
177(713), *178*(731)
Slotkin, E., 44, *49*
Smedik, P. G., 73(280), *84*(280)
Smidt, D., 166(797), *180*(797)
Smith, A. T., 258(1262), *289*(1262)
Smith, A. U., 42, *49*
Smith, B. D., 175(895), *183*(895)
Smith, B. G., 105(469), *109*(469)
Smith, G. V., 204(1004), 211(1077),
212(1077), *213*(1004), *216*(1077)
Smith, H., 75(298), 128(608), *85*
(298), *147*(608)
Smith, J. A., 285(1414), *294*(1414)
Smith, L., 231(1188), 240(1188),
235(1188)
Smith, O. W., 204(1004), 211(1075,
1077), 212(1077), *213*(1004), *216*
(1075, 1077)
Smith, P. E., 3(3), *9*(3)
Snell, G. D., 44, *50*
Snyder, F. F., 123(581), *146*(581)
Sobrero, A. J., 279(1378), *293*(1378)
Soderwall, A. L., 96(425, 426), *101*
(425, 426)
Soffer, L. J., 81(345, 346, 347, 348),
86(345, 346, 347, 348)
Soler-Bechara, J., 278(1374), *293*
(1374)
Sommers, S. C., 188(911), *195*(911)

Sonnen, N., 159(726, 727), *177*(726,
727)
Soper, E. H., 150(663), *175*(663)
Sorensen, H. B., 227(1144), *234*
(1144)
Southam, A. L., 193(949), 200(973),
211(1079), 240(1206), 279(1376,
1377), *196*(949), *212*(973), *216*
(1079), *287*(1206), *293*(1376,
1377)
Southcott, W. H., 166(794), *180*
(794)
Spaziani, E., 116(533), 157(533),
159(733), *145*(533), *178*(733)
Squier, A. H., 4(11), *9*(11)
Stamler, J., 276(1364), *292*(1364)
Stamm, O., 143(656), *149*(656)
Stanisfield, D. A., 82(358), *87*(358)
Stearns, L. W., 106(482), *109*(482)
Steelman, S. L., 74(293), 166(786),
205(1017), 209(1048), 229
(1017), *85*(293), *179*(786), *214*
(1017), *215*(1048)
Steeno, O., 268(1321), *291*(1321)
Stein, A. A., 204(998), *213*(998)
Stein, I. F., 207(1036), *214*(1036)
Stein, K., 17(66), *25*(66)
Steinberg, M., 165(782), *179*(782)
Steinberger, E., 37(147, 149), 38
(165), 39(188), 193(951), *55*
(147, 149, 165), *56*(188), *196*
(951)
Steinmetz, C. R., 14(48), *25*(48)
Stepus, S., 43, *48*
Stern, E., 263(1290), *290*(1290)
Stevens, V. C., 205(1027), 229
(1175), *214*(1027), *235*(1175)
Stewart, E. H., Jr., 44, *47*
Stob, M., 168(818), *180*(818)
Stoerk, H. C., 30(117), *54*(117)
Stoll, B. A., 259(1274), *289*(1274)
Stone, A., 210(1067), *215*(1067)
Stone, G. M., 126(589, 592), 151
(666), 154(689, 694), *147*(589,
592), *175*(666), *176*(689, 694)

Subject Index

gen-estrogen combination on, 230

stimulation of follicle to ovulation by pituitary gonadotropic hormones, 4

Ovulation

agents inhibiting, mechanisms, species differences in, 78

detection in women, 199–209
by measurement of estrogen excretion rates and blood levels, 204
of urinary and blood gonadotropin levels, 204–205
by recording and analyses of BBT, 201–202
by smear tests, 200–201
by spot color reactions, 208–209

gonadotropin dependence of ovarian follicle for, 4

induced by exogenous gonadotropin administration, 75, 77
compounds inhibiting, 76(T), 77(T), 78

inhibition of, clinical studies, 217–237
as mechanism of oral steroid contraception, 231
by steroids, 59ff
mechanism, 66
in women
by depot progestins, 231
by dithiocarbamoylhydrazine, 232

inhibitors
assay in women, 219–225
endometrial changes, 222–223
postponement of menstruation, 223–224
pregnanediol excretion, 220–221
synthetic, see also Progestin-estrogen combinations, and individual agents
control of conception and, 217, 218(T)

stimulation of, 209–212
in animals, 209
in women
by human gonadotropins, 210
by nonsteroidal agents, 210–212
by steroid hormones, 210

Ovulen, see also Contraceptives, oral and Progestin-estrogen combinations
effect on cervix, 253
on liver function, 273, 274(T)
hematological findings in users of, 278(T)
mean frequency of coitus in users of, 285, 286(T)
menstrual symptoms in users of, 303–304
reasons for discontinuing use of, 300(T)
side effects, 301(T), 304(T)

Oxytocin
inhibition of corpora lutea development, 141–142
mechanism of, 142

P

Pentose, role in cleaving egg, 108

Pheromone, urinary, in mice, 141

Phthaloyl-D-isoglutamine, as blastocyst poison, 139

Pigs, estrogen-labile pituitary LTH mechanism in, 142

Pineal gland
inhibitor of uterine and vaginal estrogen action in, 152–153

Pituitary
interrelationship with hypothalamus, 71–75
ovary and, 21
weight, effect of steroids on, 32(T)–34(T)

Pituitary hypothalamic feedback, 66

Placenta, progesterone secretion by, HCG and, 21